Welcome

It's fair to say, we could probably all do with being more present. Life is hectic, and the ever-growing number of demands and responsibilities that are placed on us can make it feel like we're in a relentless cycle of working, cooking, keeping the home tidy and flopping on the sofa. Any time out tends to be sitting in front of a screen, whether that's scrolling through social media on our phones, watching Netflix or playing video games. And while that's fine in moderation, it can mean we're missing out on everything else life has to offer: friends, family, hobbies, exercise, good food, a decent night's sleep!

Perhaps you've already created a positive work-life balance, but you've lost sight of the things you used to enjoy doing – reading a book, playing an instrument, or practising a favourite sport. Or maybe you simply feel like you're not spending quality time with the people you love.

On the pages that follow, you'll find advice and ideas on how to slow down, be present, focus and really think about what's important to you. There are interactive activities for you to complete and space for you to write down your own thoughts, as we encourage you to look at yourself, your relationships with others, your lifestyle, your mental and physical wellbeing and much more. It's time to step out of your comfort zone and start creating the life you want to live!

Contents

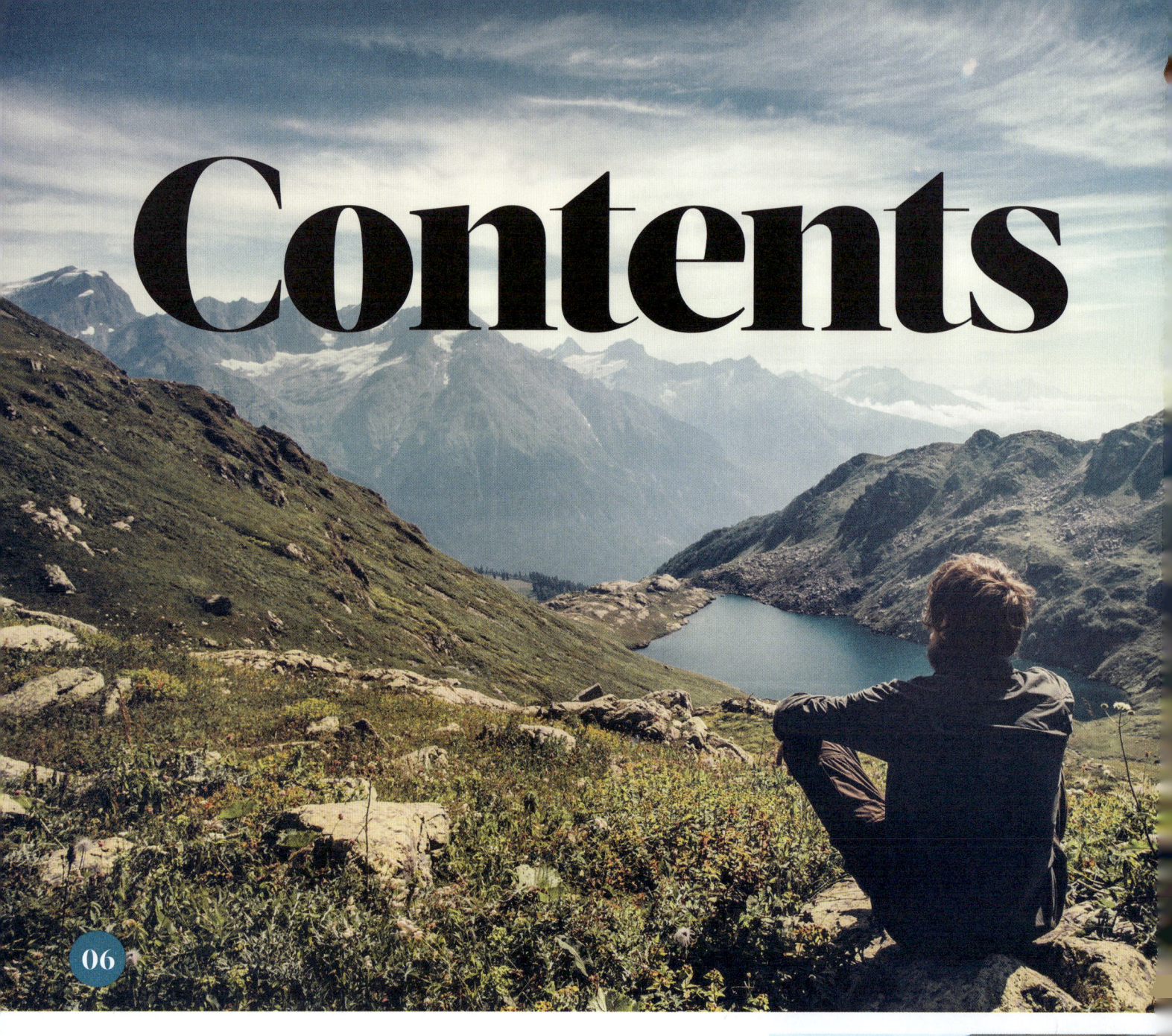

06

- 06 What is mindfulness?
- 08 Why mindfulness is beneficial
- 10 Stereotypes and expectations
- 14 Who am I?
- 20 It's a family affair
- 26 You've got a friend in me
- 30 Relationships and sex
- 36 Mindfulness in the workplace
- 42 Money makes the world go round
- 48 Hobbies and interests
- 54 A mindful work-life balance
- 60 Understanding mental health
- 68 Why it's important to talk

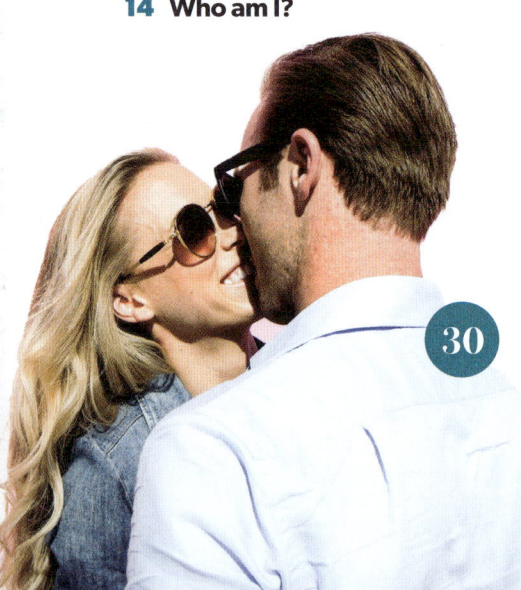

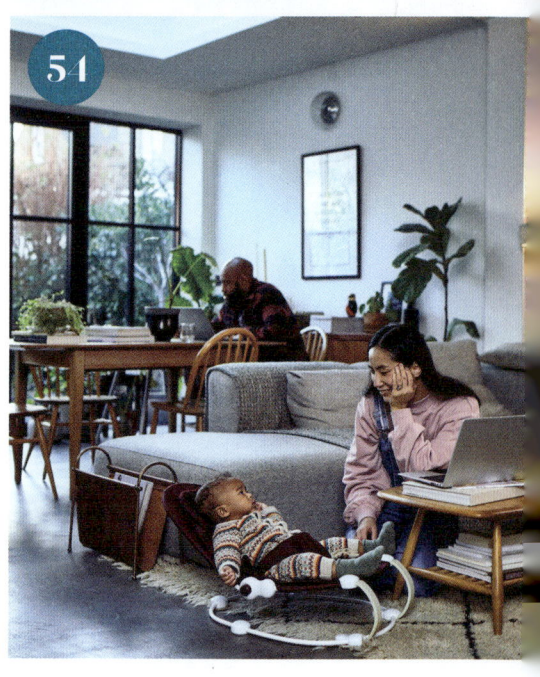

30

54

70 Learn to relax

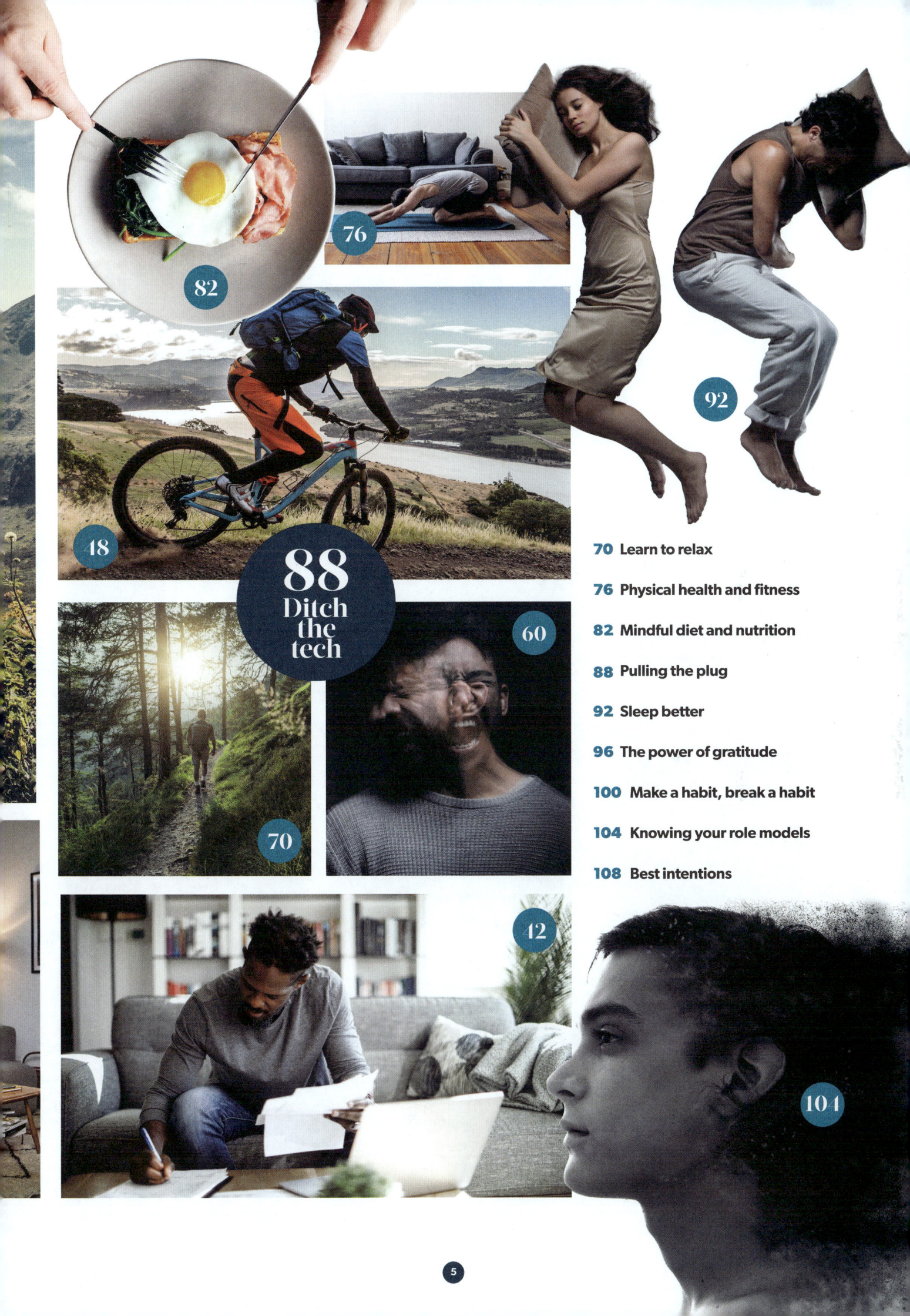

76 Physical health and fitness

82 Mindful diet and nutrition

88 Pulling the plug

92 Sleep better

96 The power of gratitude

100 Make a habit, break a habit

104 Knowing your role models

108 Best intentions

Mindfulness for Men

WHAT IS MINDFUL

TRY A GUIDED MEDITATION
If you can't still your mind and struggle to focus, an audio guided meditation app might help.

NESS?

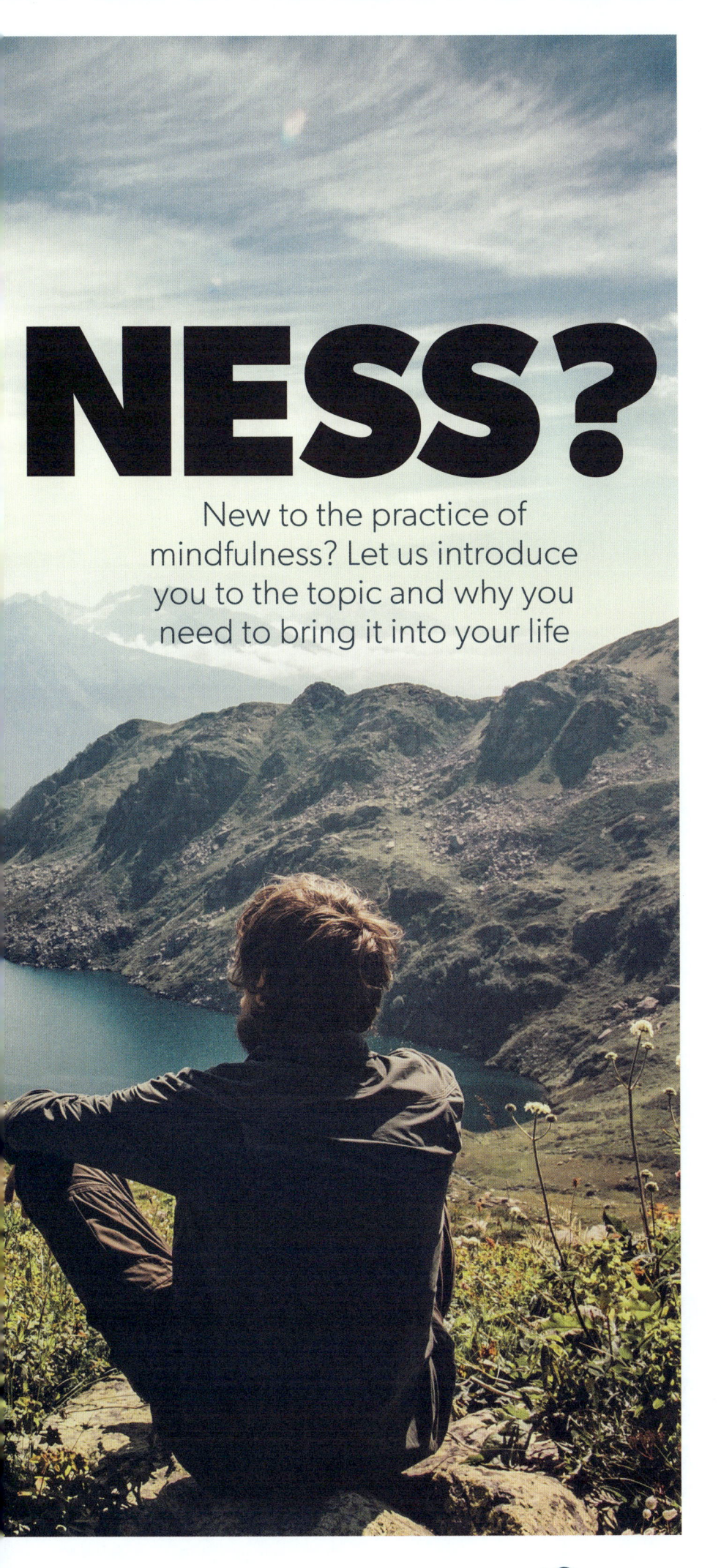

New to the practice of mindfulness? Let us introduce you to the topic and why you need to bring it into your life

What is mindfulness?

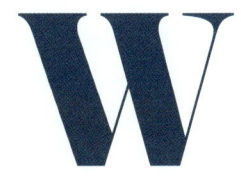

W

hen we say 'mindfulness', what does that conjure in your mind? Long meditations, yoga sessions and daily journalling? Well, yes, it can be those things for some people, but that's just a handful of ways to practise mindfulness, and it doesn't have to look anything like that if that's not right for you.

Mindfulness can help to improve your mental health, your overall wellbeing, your stress responses, your relationships, your concentration and memory, and so much more. We have dedicated pages to the benefits of mindfulness in the next section, where we'll go into this in more detail, but first, we're looking to understand what mindfulness is.

To be mindful is to be aware and present in the moment, no matter what you're doing. It's about noticing your surroundings, not just letting them pass you by. It's being aware of your thoughts and feelings, without judgement, and acknowledging them. It's about fully engaging in what you're doing without distraction.

If you feel like you're rushing through life, often feeling busy and stressed, a little disconnected and unmotivated, mindfulness might help. It can embolden you to become more aware about the way you live your life, and encourage you to take the time to get more out of the things you do.

You don't need to be mindful all the time. It's about introducing it into your life bit by bit. You might want to start with a dedicated mindfulness practice during your day for a few minutes, before applying it to other areas of your life. The simplest way to do this is to sit comfortably in silence with your thoughts. Notice your breath as it goes in and out, notice the thoughts that come into your mind, notice the feelings you have, notice how your body feels. It can be difficult at first – your mind might wander, or you might feel a bit silly. But gently try to bring your focus back to your thoughts and feelings in that moment.

If you find sitting still just too hard, you can try a walking meditation instead. Rather than just walking to go from A to B, without paying attention to the journey, try walking with purpose. Look at the things around you as you walk, noticing the little details. What can you hear, smell, touch and see?

Once you've mastered these basic techniques, you're ready to start thinking about how to bring more mindfulness into your life, and reap the many rewards.

Mindfulness for Men

WHY MINDFULNESS IS BENEFICIAL

Understanding the potential benefits can help you to make more time for mindfulness in your life

Becoming more mindful, whether that's through specific relaxation activities and meditation, or approaching your usual hobbies and exercise in a more mindful way, can have a huge number of benefits.

Maybe you're completely new to mindfulness, or maybe you've tried before but given up too soon. Or maybe you're already aware of the benefits of mindfulness and you're looking to improve and increase your practice of it. Whatever brought you to this point and made you pick up this book, you must have some level of interest in mindfulness to have made that purchase.

Living a more mindful life can lead to living a happier, more fulfilled life. Mindfulness has huge benefits for everyone, regardless of gender, but a lot of the mindfulness resources available online are targeted towards women, which can make it seem inaccessible. And yet, the majority of monks who regularly practise mindfulness and meditation are men, who extol the virtues of leading a more mindful life. It is slowly becoming more mainstream, with sports brands like ASICS running campaigns around mindfulness, and tech companies such as Apple building meditation and mindfulness into their products. If you wear a smartwatch, you might find that this has handy features around mindfulness too.

Some of the general benefits include an improvement in overall wellbeing, reduced stress, better focus and concentration, and improved mental health. Some small-scale studies have suggested that the way men and women process emotions is different; women are more likely to internally process emotions and ruminate over them, whereas men can be better at externally processing emotions, by doing physical activity or playing a videogame, for example. These are sweeping generalisations of course. Mindfulness can help you to become more aware of your thoughts, emotions and feelings. It can give you the tools to confront these, and the techniques to help control them. Mindful practice can also help you to reduce workplace- and home-related anxiety and stress, particularly with regular opportunities to relax and engage in hobbies.

Mindfulness can also help increase self-compassion, and let go of societal expectations. This, in itself, can improve mental health and wellbeing, and enable you to live a more authentic lifestyle. If you start meditating, you certainly won't be alone. A US-based study[1] found that between 2012 and 2017, the number of people who reported meditating more than tripled.

Meditation and mindfulness can be beneficial to those with certain health conditions, including inflammatory conditions like IBS or ulcerative colitis, anxiety and depression, stress and insomnia. It can also be a helpful tool for those who want to stop smoking or reduce their alcohol intake by offering a distraction and relaxation. There are also small studies that suggest meditation could help with male infertility, lower blood pressure and regulate hormones, though there is no solid medical evidence for these. Living a healthier, calmer lifestyle that includes mindful practice will certainly help boost mental and physical health.

If you do have any mental or physical health conditions, it is worth consulting with a doctor before starting something new. Some of the suggestions in this book are not suitable for everyone – for example, yoga might not be appropriate for some people with physical health conditions, and intense breathwork should be approached cautiously by those with asthma, for example, or other lung conditions.

1. Use of Yoga, Meditation, and Chiropractors Among U.S. Adults Aged 18 and Over, November 2018, Tainya C Clarke et al

Inspirational role models

These motivational men can help you get to grips with the benefits of mindfulness and meditation

JAY SHETTY
www.jayshetty.me

At the age of 21, after hearing a monk speak and feeling inspired, Jay Shetty began to live a split life, working half of his summer vacations in finance and the other half living as a monk in India. After three years, he committed to life with the monks, living there for the next three years to focus on self-growth. On his return, he worked towards his life's purpose: sharing the wisdom he had gained as a monk, and encouraging everyone to find their purpose and live more mindfully.

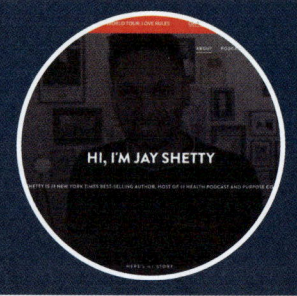

HI, I'M JAY SHETTY

Why mindfulness is beneficial

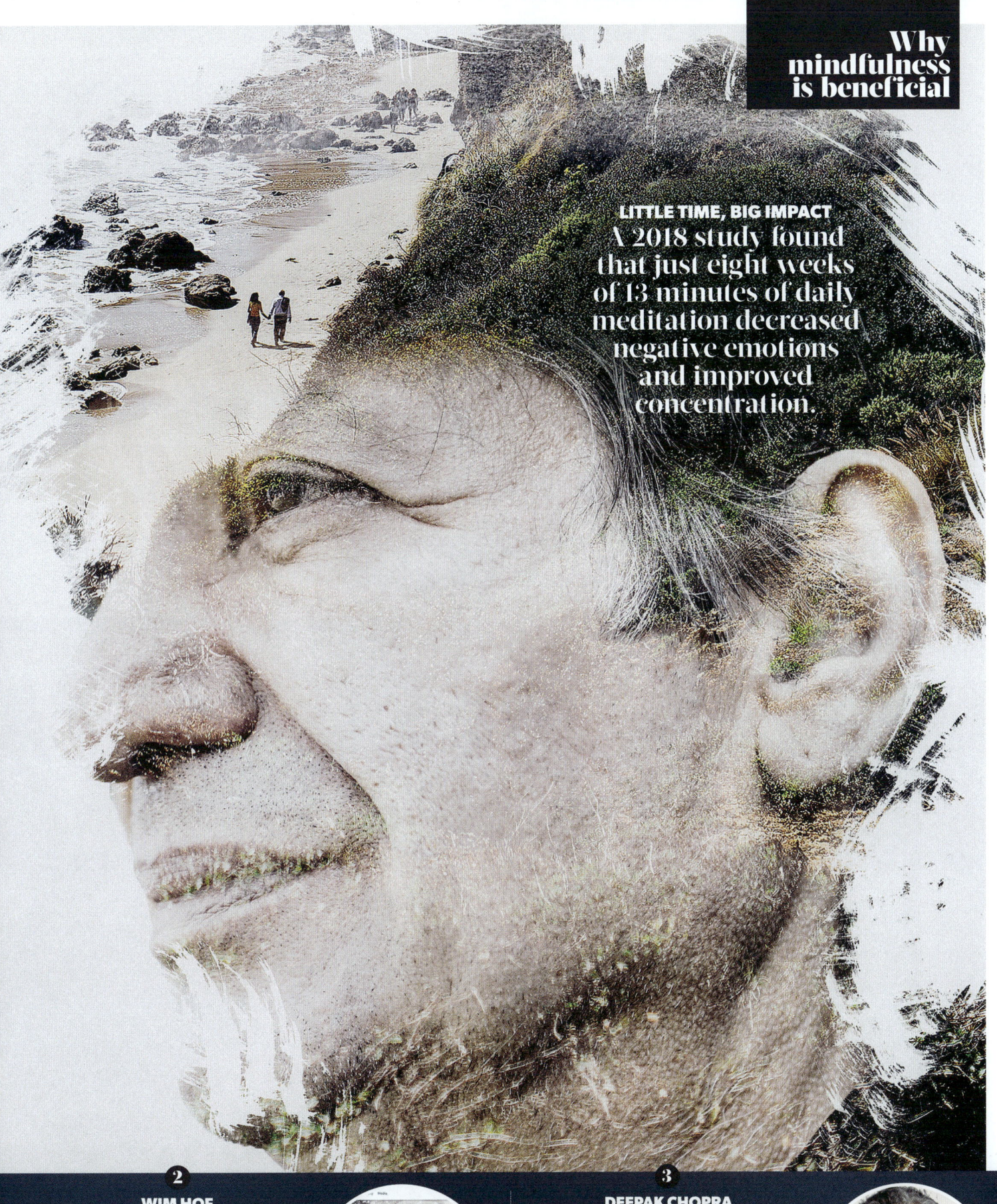

LITTLE TIME, BIG IMPACT
A 2018 study found that just eight weeks of 13 minutes of daily meditation decreased negative emotions and improved concentration.

2
WIM HOF
www.wimhofmethod.com
You've probably heard of Wim Hof and associate him with ice baths, but his practice goes much deeper than that, teaching you how to optimise your mind and body in their natural states. Yes, part of this is cold therapy, but it also includes breathing techniques and commitment.

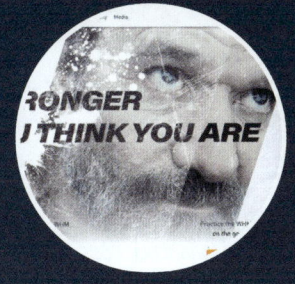

3
DEEPAK CHOPRA
www.deepakchopra.com
One of the best-known names in meditation, Chopra has written more than 90 books, translated into more than 43 languages. *TIME* magazine described him as one of the top 100 heroes and icons of the century. His books and resources can teach you how to unlock your potential and live your life with purpose.

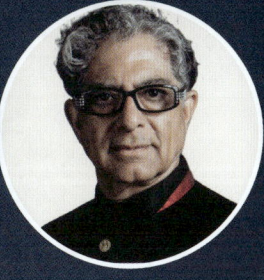

Navigating female dominated spaces

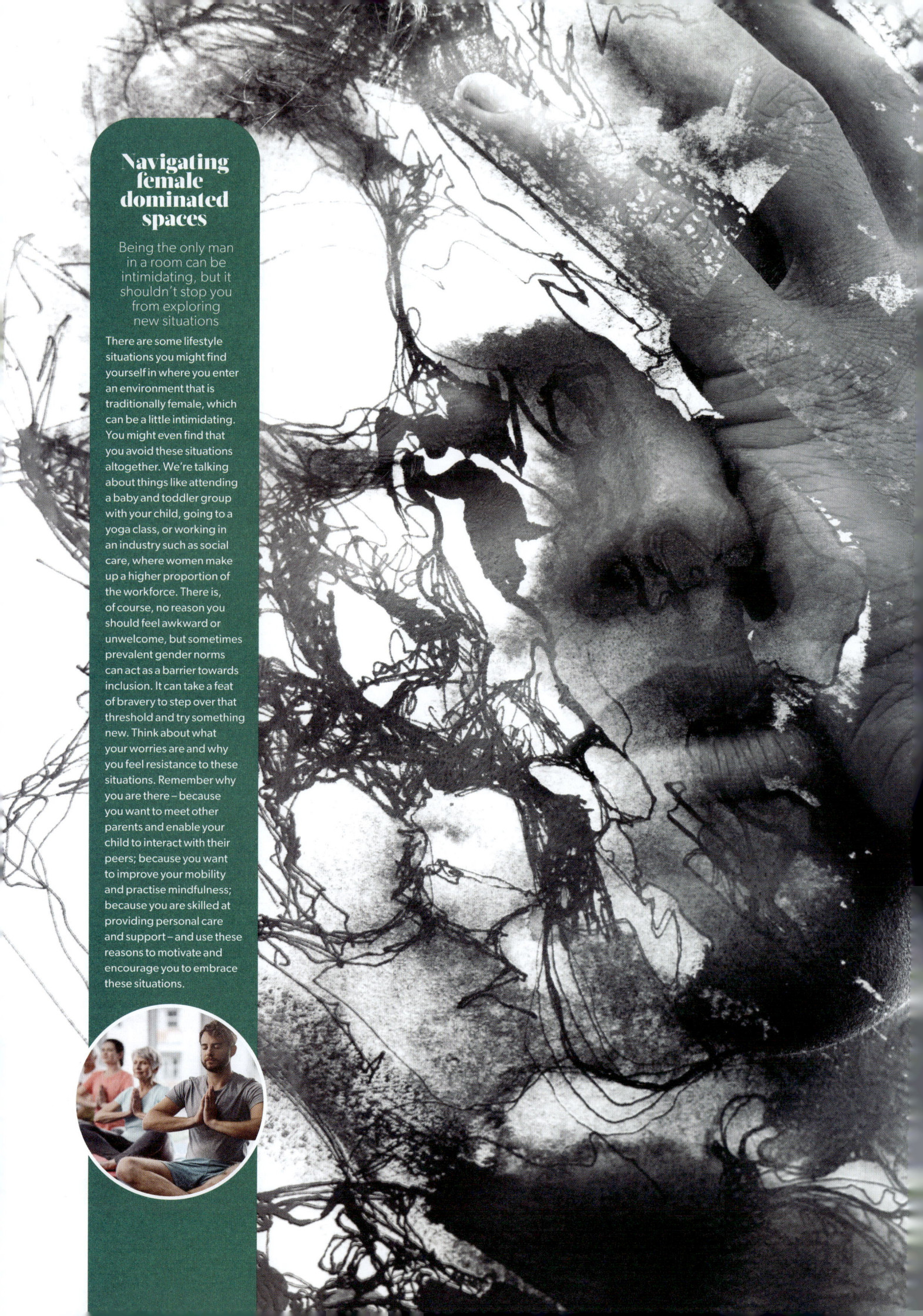

Being the only man in a room can be intimidating, but it shouldn't stop you from exploring new situations

There are some lifestyle situations you might find yourself in where you enter an environment that is traditionally female, which can be a little intimidating. You might even find that you avoid these situations altogether. We're talking about things like attending a baby and toddler group with your child, going to a yoga class, or working in an industry such as social care, where women make up a higher proportion of the workforce. There is, of course, no reason you should feel awkward or unwelcome, but sometimes prevalent gender norms can act as a barrier towards inclusion. It can take a feat of bravery to step over that threshold and try something new. Think about what your worries are and why you feel resistance to these situations. Remember why you are there – because you want to meet other parents and enable your child to interact with their peers; because you want to improve your mobility and practise mindfulness; because you are skilled at providing personal care and support – and use these reasons to motivate and encourage you to embrace these situations.

STEREOTYPES AND EXPECTATIONS

Stereotypes and expectations

Why it's important to be aware of the pressures and challenges that unhelpful stereotypes can present – and how to overcome them

We're all exposed to gender-based stereotypes, often on a daily basis, whether we're aware of it or not. It starts early in life – from the day we're born, in fact. Clothes for newborn babies can be found neatly in their own sections for 'boys' and 'girls' – which might be perfectly understandable if the clothing was specifically designed to address sex-based differences in male and female bodies, but actually, in most cases, it offers simply a different choice of colour and pattern.

It doesn't get better as you get older either: dark, practical colours and hardwearing materials for the boys; pastels, leggings and dresses for the girls. Toys, too, are often split along gender lines in shops, and well-meaning relatives may have gifted differently for male and female children. At school, uniforms mark clear differences between the genders; at playtimes, football is for the boys and netball is for the girls.

These are just a few examples of the types of stereotypes you may have experienced up to this point in your life. It might be that you've never consciously considered these aspects of your childhood and teenage years. We are all driven by an innate need to be accepted and to 'fit in' when we're growing up, meaning we never stop to question these unhelpful and often dangerous gender stereotypes.

SOCIETAL EXPECTATIONS
This level of bias and stereotyping is harmful, which is something that we're only really starting to explore in today's world. These deeply ingrained societal expectations and beliefs put a lot of pressure on men. We've been told – whether overtly or via representations of men in the media – what is expected of us. To be tough, to not show emotion, to be strong, to provide, to protect... the list goes on. And with this comes a lot of pressure. If you spend a whole life growing up being taught that you need to behave in one way, what happens when you don't?

For one thing, it can have a huge impact on your wellbeing. These gender stereotypes around masculinity carry huge risks around poor mental health. Men are, in many cases, less encouraged to talk about feelings, emotions and stresses, which means that they're more inclined to hold these in, or use less healthy coping mechanisms (such as drinking more alcohol than usual, getting angry, and so on). We explore more about mental health and talking to others elsewhere in this book, so do take the time to read those features. Despite what gender stereotypes might try to persuade us otherwise, it's really healthy to show true emotions – it's the body's way of coping in difficult situations. Crying, feeling angry or getting frustrated are all normal outlets for our emotions, and it's far healthier for our mental state to allow these feelings out.

BATTLING THE STIGMA
Another issue is that these 'gender norms' can create stigma around perfectly normal feelings, actions, relationships and lifestyles, which can make us ask questions or deny those things that would make us happier. For example, when it comes to having children, the societal norm is for the mother to stay at home, while the father goes out to work. This may work fine for some families, but by presenting it as the 'normal' or 'ideal' way of doing things disregards the many other family set-ups that might work much better in your own situation. What if your family isn't made up that way? You may be in a same-sex relationship and have made the decision to have children together. You might be in a relationship where the mother of your children earns more money or wants to return to work full-

CRYING BY GENDER
Men cry emotional tears 5 to 17 times a year, in comparison to 30 to 64 times a year for women[1].

1. 'Country and Crying: Prevalences and Gender Differences', van Hemert et al, 2011

Mindfulness for Men

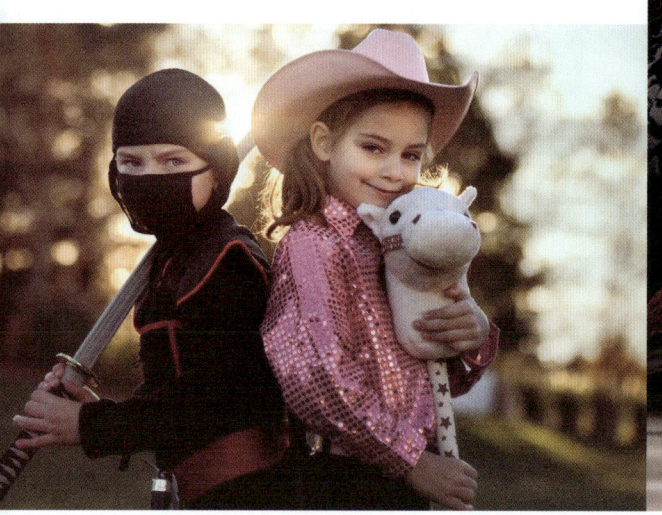

CALL IT OUT
Don't be afraid to question others when they make gender assumptions or enforce expectations.

Above: From clothing to toys, children are taught from a young age that they should play or dress a certain way

Below: Although it's gradually becoming better, male- and female-dominated spaces still exist; whether for work or play

time, meaning it makes sense for you to be the parent who stays at home with your baby. If your situation is different from what society has traditionally considered 'normal', it can feel like the world isn't set up with the tools and resources to help you navigate family life, which subconsciously reinforces the stigma, and in turn has an impact on your mental health and wellbeing.

According to law firm EMW, in 2020-2021 in the UK, paternity leave hit a ten-year low, and in 2022 only a third of eligible new fathers took their paternity leave. This was fuelled by the low rates of Statutory Paternity Pay being offered by the government, as well as many companies not offering a policy to allow fathers to take the time off they need to play an active role in important early months and years of a child's life. It's no better in the USA; although fathers are entitled to 12 weeks of paternity leave, this is unpaid, making it impractical for most families to manage. Coupled with the pressure of being seen as a 'provider' and the stigma imposed on men who choose to spend time away from the workplace to be with their children, it can be very difficult to make that decision to do what's right for you and not what's deemed right by outdated and archaic views.

TAKING POSITIVE ACTION
So, what can we do in the face of these stereotypes and expectations, which seem to be built in to the fabric of our society? Things are starting to change – the tide is turning on old-fashioned gender expectations. There is meaningful conversation happening around the damage that gender stereotypes can cause, and extreme examples of toxic masculinity are being called out. The first

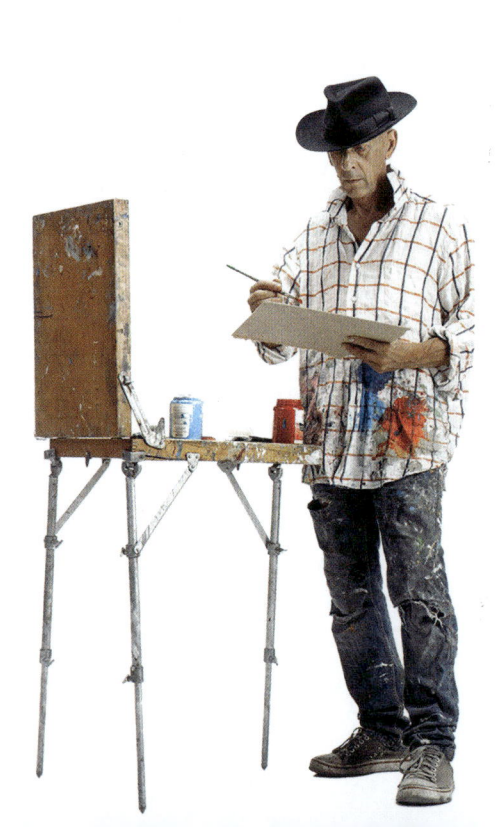

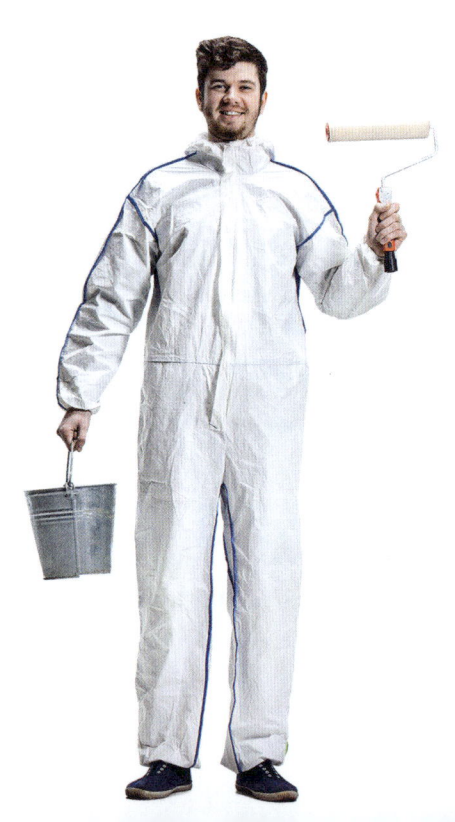

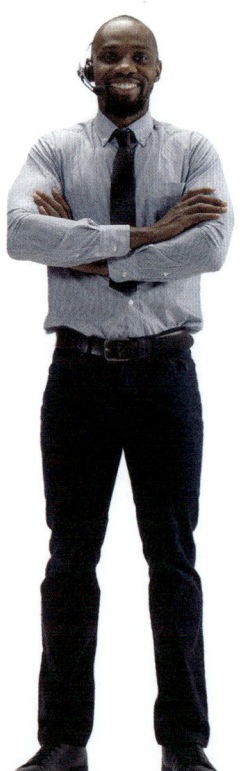

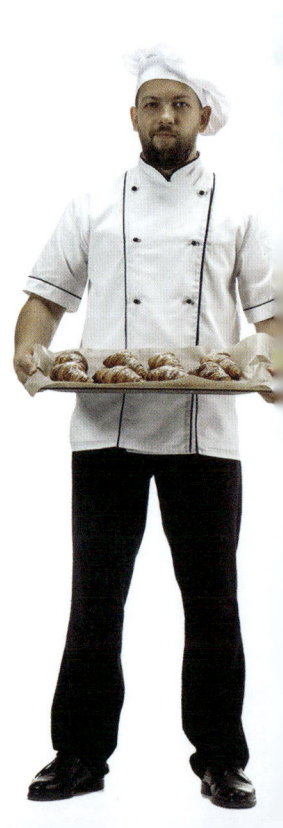

Stereotypes and expectations

When we begin to recognise these feelings, we can start to work on overcoming them. Rather than acting in a way that feels 'right' based on what you think you 'should' do, think instead about what you 'want' and what would make you happy. The more that you make decisions based on what's right for you and the people in your life, the happier and more content you will be. Throughout this book, we explore many different areas of your life, from your hobbies and how you relax, to your relationships and your work-life balance. Every one of these areas can be impacted by deep-set beliefs around gender stereotypes – we encourage you to explore what really makes you happy or relaxed, or what you enjoy. Gently push away any intruding thoughts and feelings you encounter that may try to dissuade you, but recognise these feelings as this will help you to understand some of the bias you might have absorbed throughout your life without consciously realising.

Below: These days, there's thankfully no such thing as a 'typical' family set-up

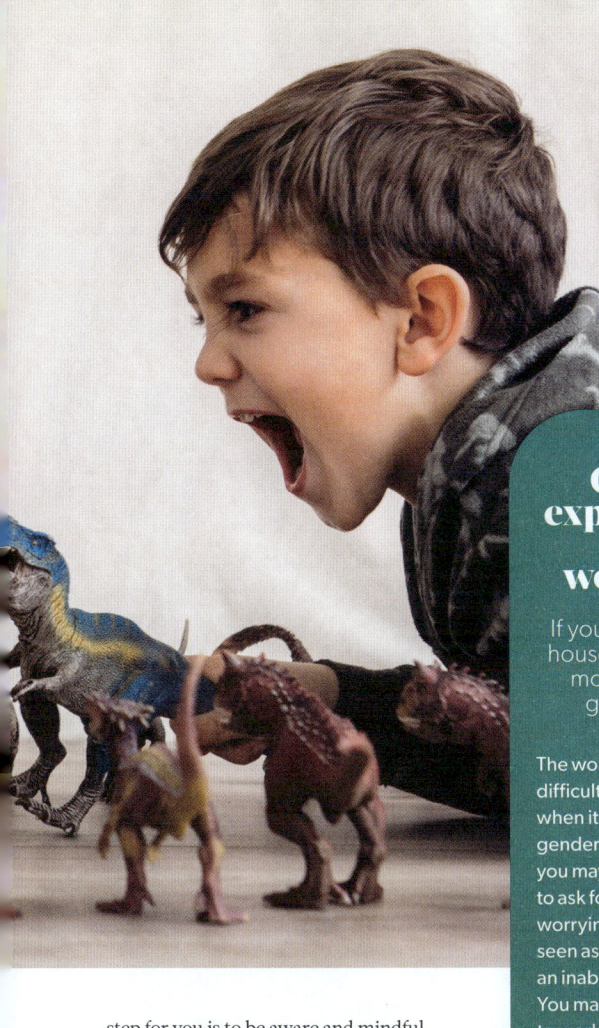

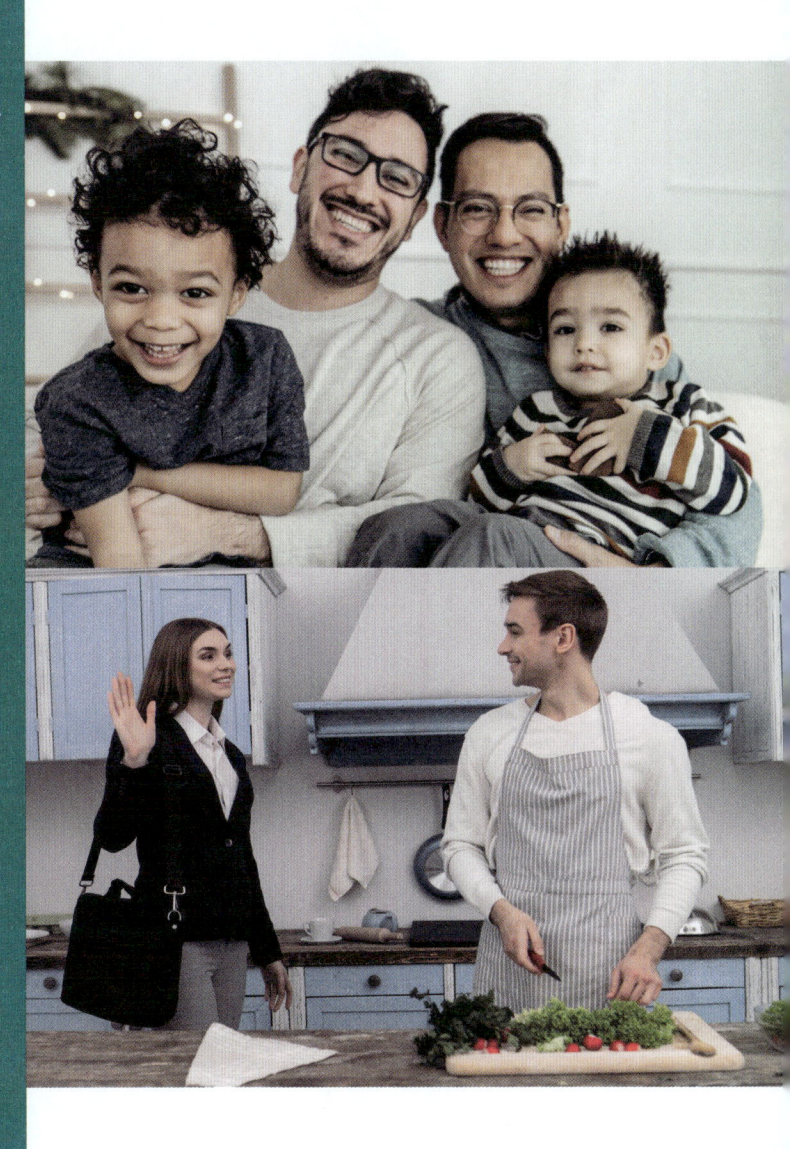

step for you is to be aware and mindful of these stereotypes and consider how they might be impacting your life, your thoughts and your feelings. Allow yourself time to think about areas in your life where you feel a pressure to behave or live in a certain way. Why do you think you feel that way? Where do those feelings come from? You might feel a mental resistance around certain actions – for example, you might refrain from talking about something that is worrying you – so when you feel that, try to explore your feelings, and think about where that opposition is coming from.

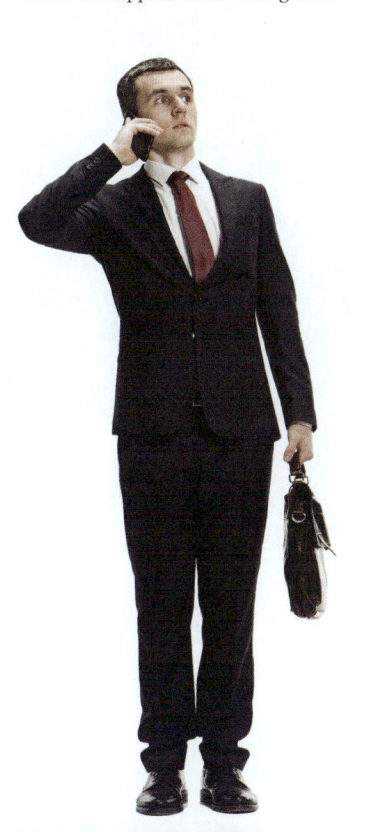

Gender expectations in the workplace

If you work out of the house, you might feel more exposed to gender-based pressures

The workplace can be a difficult place to navigate when it comes to ingrained gender norms. As a man, you may find it more difficult to ask for help, for example, worrying that this could be seen as weak or show up an inability to do your job. You may also feel a pressure to work longer hours and spend time in networking situations when you'd rather be at home. Or you might find that you act a different way with your colleagues than you would do in your day-to-day life.

The problem is that many of these stereotypes are built in to the fabric of work life, and it can be very difficult to suddenly begin to implement change. Identify areas in which you would like to make adjustments that reflect who you are as a person, and be mindful about how you can do this sensitively. It might be that you want to start leaving the office on time, but are worried about doing so if you're in an environment where everyone stays late. You could start by leaving five minutes earlier, and then ten, and so on. You may even encourage those around you to do the same – it's often the case that many men feel the same, but are all trapped, afraid of the same stigma, and sometimes it takes just one person to do something differently to adjust the situation.

Mindfulness for Men

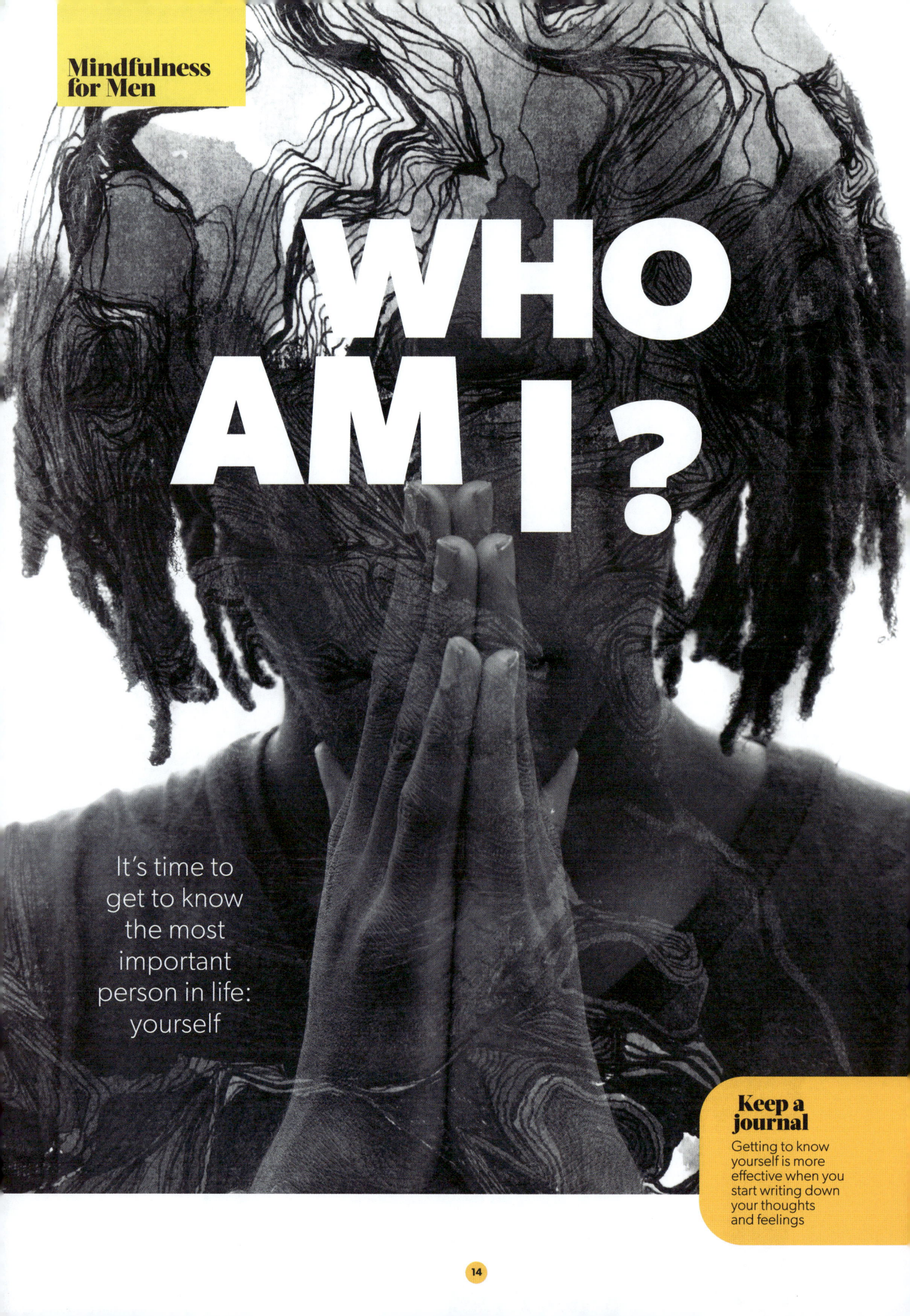

WHO AM I?

It's time to get to know the most important person in life: yourself

Keep a journal
Getting to know yourself is more effective when you start writing down your thoughts and feelings

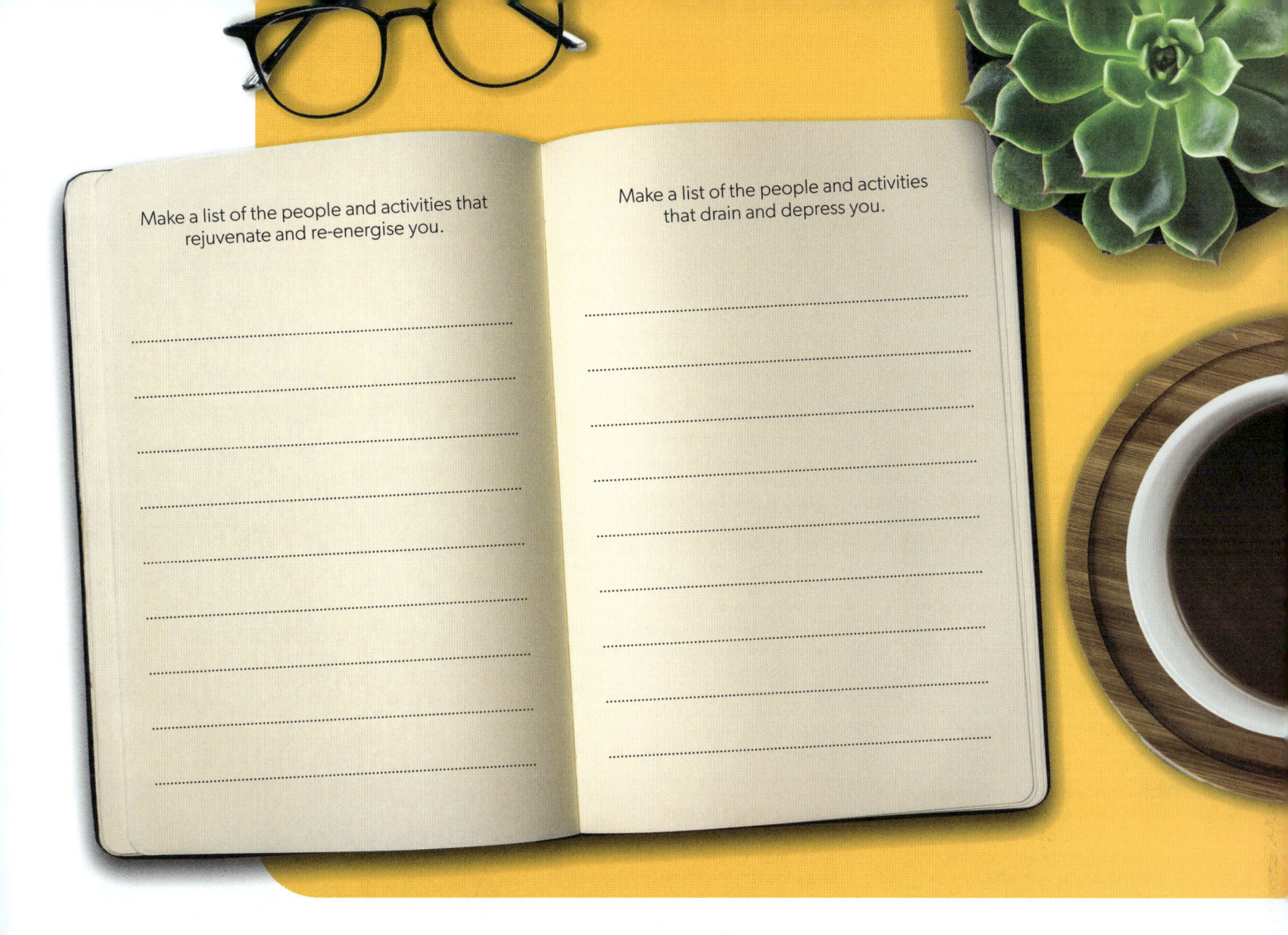

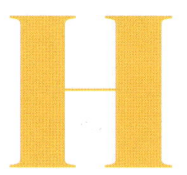

Make a list of the people and activities that rejuvenate and re-energise you.

Make a list of the people and activities that drain and depress you.

How well do you know yourself? It may sound like an odd question, but there are different levels to each one of us. You may feel your sense of self is wrapped up in the work you do and the career you have pursued. You may feel your sense of self is reflected in the books you read, the movies you watch, the video games you play and the sports you follow.

But that's not truly you. To get to know yourself better entails going deeper. Indeed, it was Dogen Zenji who told us, 'to know yourself is to forget yourself', while Socrates said, 'to know thyself is the beginning of wisdom'. Those phrases might sound conflicting, but they involve paying attention to your current experiences and better understanding your feelings.

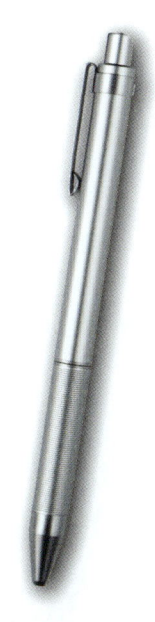

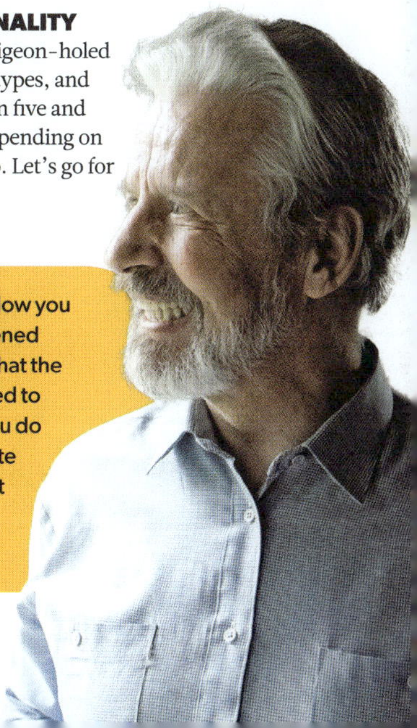

By taking the time to get to know yourself, you will learn so much about why you behave and think in the way that you do. Greater self-knowledge means you will have a better handle on your motivations, core values and beliefs. If you find yourself getting angry in a situation, for example, you will be able to work out why you are feeling that way. Your thought patterns become clearer and more consistent, and you can feel more in control.

Being a man isn't easy. You are many different things to lots of different people, and the way you interact and behave with others may, at times, frustrate you. You may ask yourself why you are feeling and behaving in the way you do as a father, a son, a brother, a husband, a boyfriend, a friend and so on. There will also be triggers that spark undesired behaviours and you may not be aware of what they are.

With self-awareness and self-knowledge, you can form better relationships with those around you, understanding how your emotions, experiences and feelings shape your interactions. You can recognise anxiety, anger and sadness in yourself, for example, and identify those triggers so that you can react more appropriately to situations, and make informed and responsible decisions. Self-awareness and self-knowledge are also likely to lead to greater empathy and understanding for others. And it all starts with you.

YOUR PERSONALITY
Men tend to be pigeon-holed into personality types, and there are between five and seven of these depending on who you listen to. Let's go for

It's easier to get to know yourself if you pick up a pen and paper and start writing things down. It is even preferable to typing your thoughts on a computer, since using a pen offers fewer distractions and it feels more intimate. After all, it's just you and a blank piece of paper, ready to be filled. You could even draw or doodle if that better helps you to express how you feel. The main thing is that you're laying down conscious knowledge of your character and feelings.

Journalling can take place any time, or it could be a reflective exercise at night. Either way, you need to reflect on your experiences and what happened to your body at those times. If we were pushed to suggest a perfect time, we'd say it's often best to reflect immediately so that you can really focus on yourself. This will allow you to more easily identify what happened before those feelings emerged, what the feelings did to you, how you wanted to react and how you did react. As you do so, rate how happy you are and note your energy levels. Reflect on what you did to resolve the situation or whether the problem still exists.

Mindfulness for Men

a middle ground of six, meaning you may be identified as an alpha, beta, gamma, omega, delta or sigma male. Once placed into such a group, your natural tendencies, likes, dislikes and habits are said to be easily explained, but are they really reflective of who you actually are?

Many of you will know what an alpha male is: someone charismatic, charming, sociable, confident, and good at leading and making decisions. Sigma males are more solitary, treat everyone equally, and seek deep connections. Beta males are eager to please, hate conflict and work hard. Delta males are shaped by experience and find it hard to trust, while gamma males are a mix of the others, and they are also self-aware while being sensitive to criticism and praise. Omega males care little about getting validation from others, and they're confident in their own abilities.

But how do you know where you fit among these personality types if you don't actually know yourself as well as you'd like? The answer is to overcome the barriers that are preventing you from learning more about yourself. One of these barriers is the overwhelming need among many men to be seen in a desirable manner. It's quite natural to want to be liked and admired, but it can cloud who you really are.

If you're trying to present virtuous qualities to boost your self-esteem or overcome negative feelings, for example, then, according to psychological scientist Erika Carlson of Washington University in St Louis, you're not getting to know yourself properly. You're using behaviour to mask your feelings. But if you're better aware of why you may have low self-esteem and are feeling negative, and you can assess this in a non-judgemental way, you will feel more confident and start to see yourself and your behaviour with greater clarity.

Carlson also says it's important to gather as much information about yourself as possible, and not having that to hand means you don't get a full sense of you. Being in tune with how your body reacts to situations, for example, can help you to gain a better understanding. Have you ever been in a meeting and wondered why your boss has started to become agitated with you? It may be because your face is giving off signs of displeasure or you look as if your mind has drifted away. Self-awareness would ensure you could control those outward signs.

ASSESS YOUR NEEDS

As you begin to assess your emotions and feelings in a given situation in a non-judgemental manner, you become more aware of your own needs, and you can begin to articulate them with clarity. You will still have worries – problems don't magically go away – but, with more self-awareness, you will understand why you are reacting to them in the way you do, and you can lessen the anxiety you feel. In short, you can respond rather than react to life events.

TAKE AN ONLINE PERSONALITY TEST

There are lots of free online personality tests. Ideally, try tests based on different theories of personality, including Myers-Briggs, Big 5 Personality, Minnesota Multiphasic Personality Inventory (MMPI) and NERIS Type Explorer.

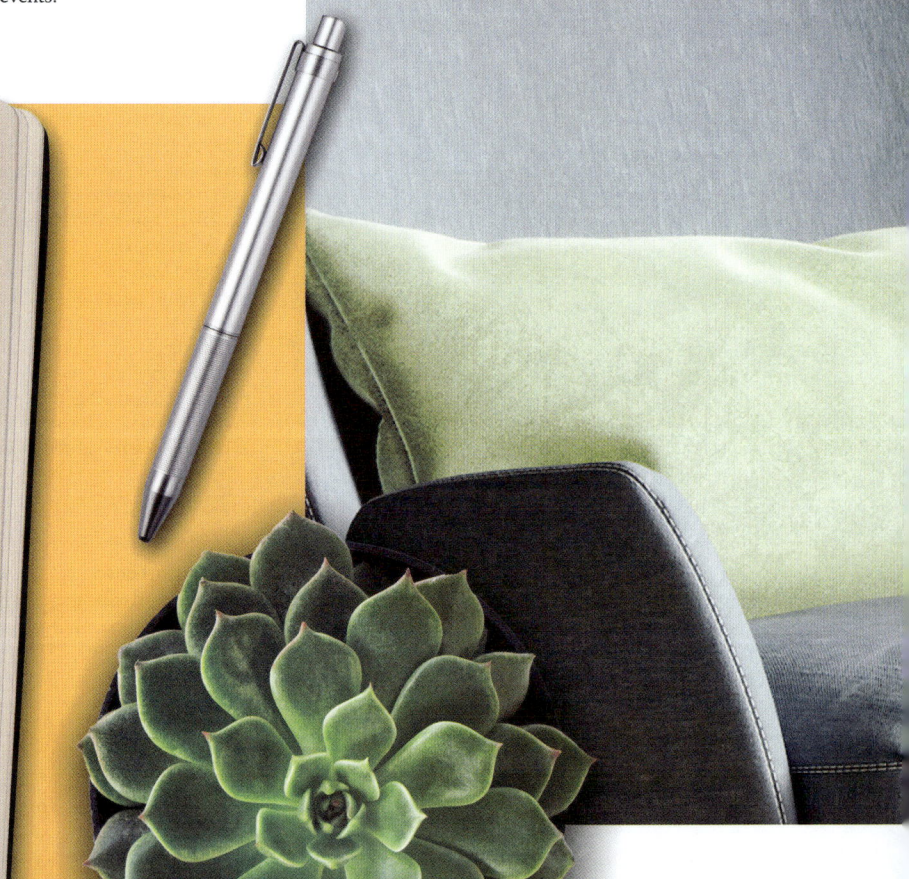

Write down here the various roles you carry out, and then number them according to their importance to you.

....
....
....
....
....
....
....

The VITALS path to self-knowledge

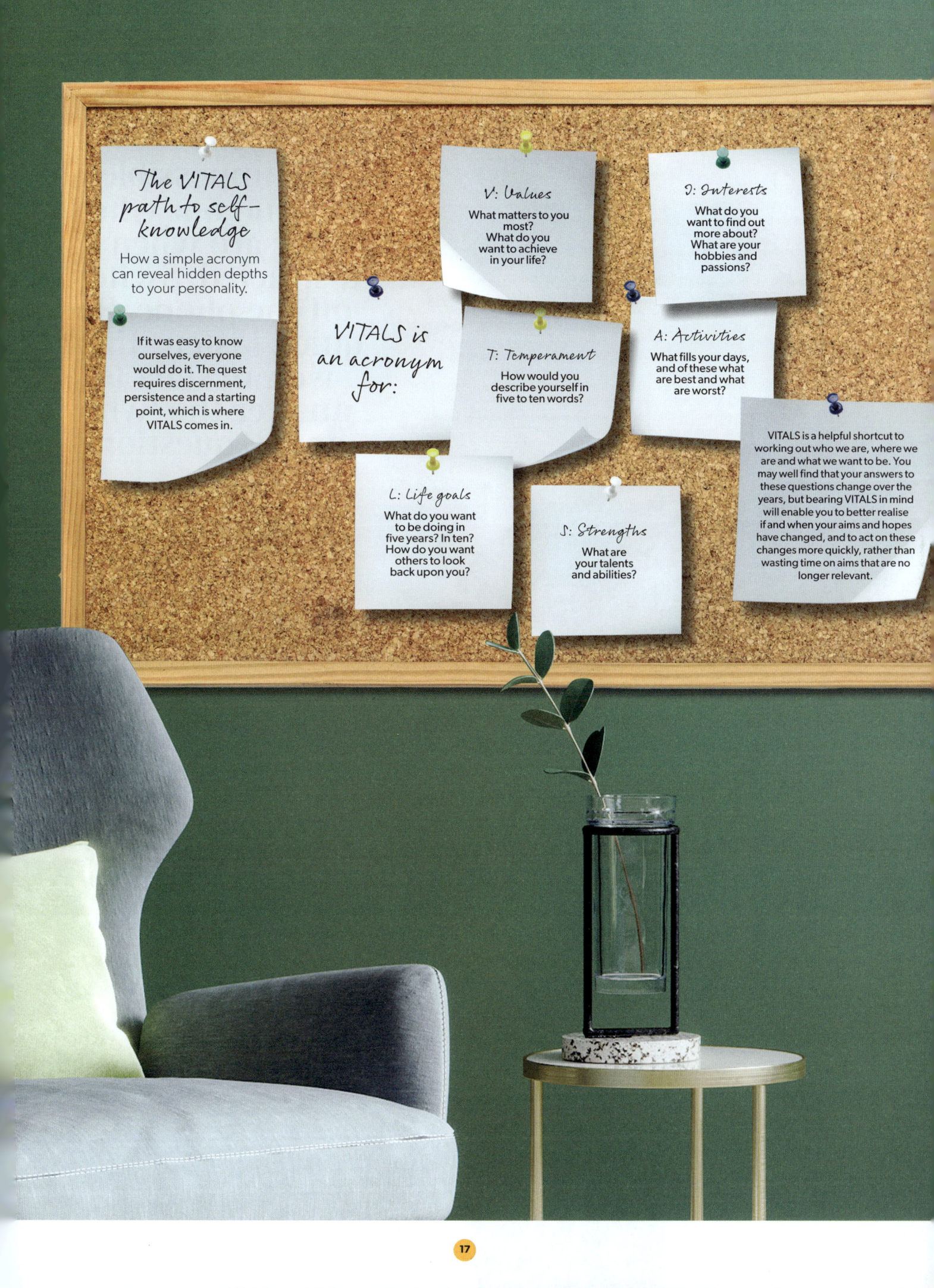

How a simple acronym can reveal hidden depths to your personality.

If it was easy to know ourselves, everyone would do it. The quest requires discernment, persistence and a starting point, which is where VITALS comes in.

VITALS is an acronym for:

V: Values
What matters to you most? What do you want to achieve in your life?

I: Interests
What do you want to find out more about? What are your hobbies and passions?

T: Temperament
How would you describe yourself in five to ten words?

A: Activities
What fills your days, and of these what are best and what are worst?

L: Life goals
What do you want to be doing in five years? In ten? How do you want others to look back upon you?

S: Strengths
What are your talents and abilities?

VITALS is a helpful shortcut to working out who we are, where we are and what we want to be. You may well find that your answers to these questions change over the years, but bearing VITALS in mind will enable you to better realise if and when your aims and hopes have changed, and to act on these changes more quickly, rather than wasting time on aims that are no longer relevant.

Mindfulness for Men

Doing so means your decision-making becomes more thoughtful because one of the effects of self-awareness is getting to know your core values and connecting with them. By understanding if you're fundamentally adventurous, balanced, bold, compassionate, competent, fun, honest, knowledgeable, loyal, open, peaceful, successful or wise, or if you have integrity, respect, responsibilities or a competitive nature, then you can identify your boundaries and become less influenced by events.

In other words, your boss may criticise you but you might know deep down that it was unwarranted and untrue so you won't be negatively affected (and if the criticism is correct then you could have the self-awareness to respond well). If someone asks you to do something dishonest, your core values will keep you true to yourself. Emotions will be less likely to dictate your life and cause you to snap at friends or avoid doing something exciting because someone believes you will fail. You will know what has triggered your anger and you will know that you have the resources to succeed.

The upshot is that you will be able to create a life that feels more satisfying and meaningful and, with self-awareness can come self-esteem and self-compassion. How you see yourself and how others see you will alter when you get to know yourself. Indeed, your identity is not fixed – it changes because people evolve. With mindfulness enabling greater self-awareness, you can allow yourself to grow.

STOP
It's impossible to find out who we are when distracted. Switch off the phone. Be quiet. Listen. Then we can start to answer the 'who am I?' question.

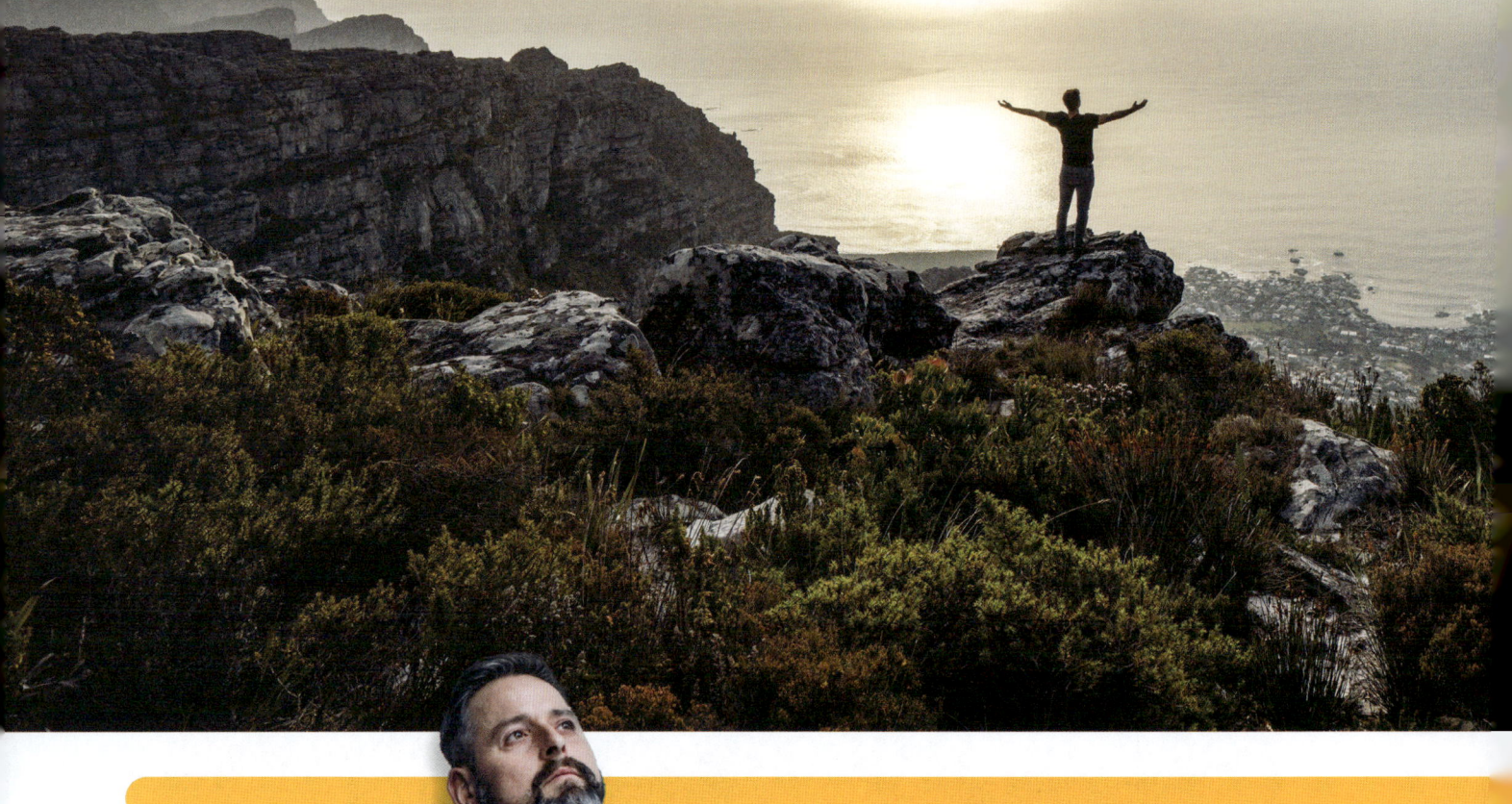

In the three goals write your goals for:

Next year

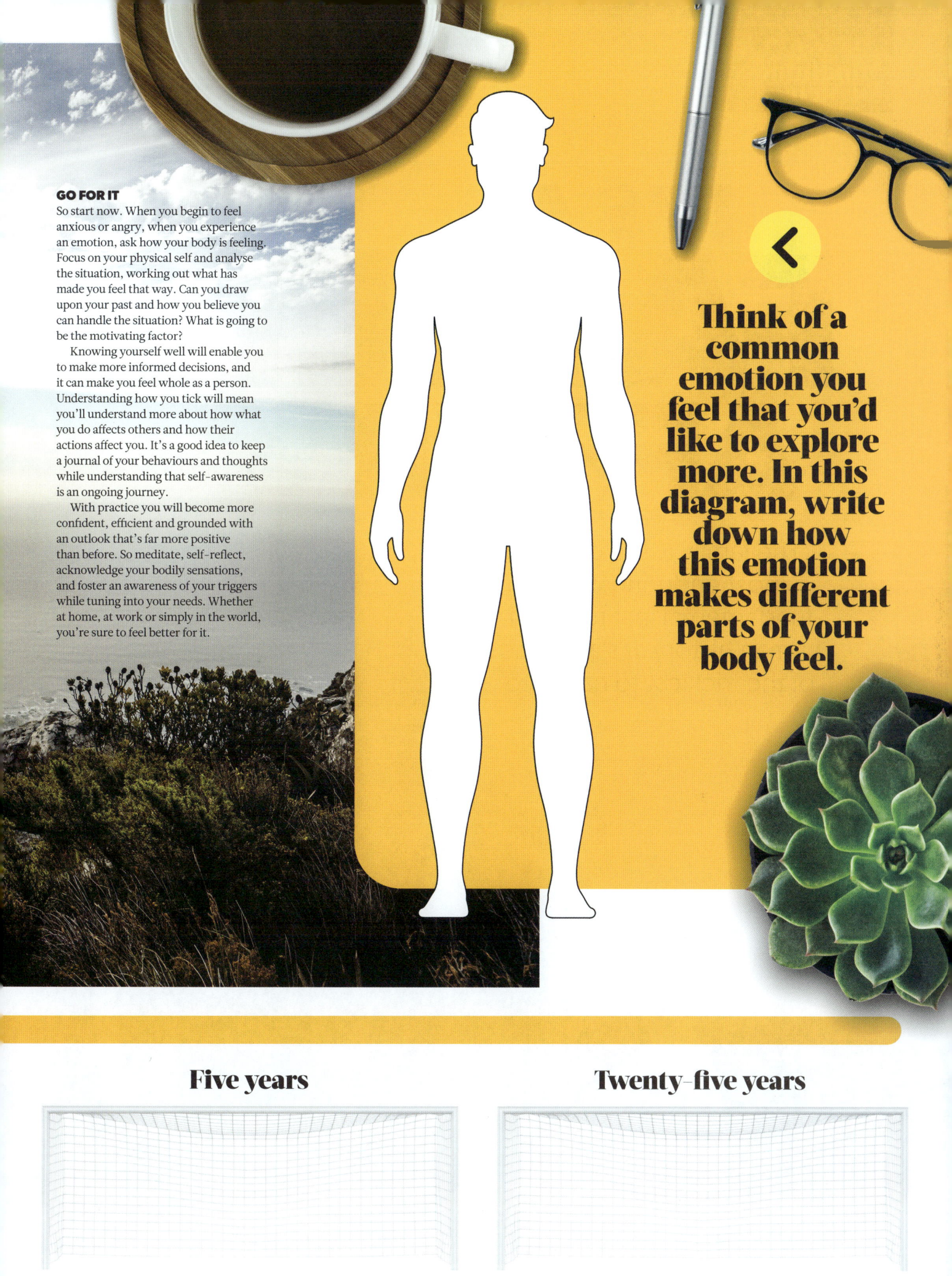

GO FOR IT
So start now. When you begin to feel anxious or angry, when you experience an emotion, ask how your body is feeling. Focus on your physical self and analyse the situation, working out what has made you feel that way. Can you draw upon your past and how you believe you can handle the situation? What is going to be the motivating factor?

Knowing yourself well will enable you to make more informed decisions, and it can make you feel whole as a person. Understanding how you tick will mean you'll understand more about how what you do affects others and how their actions affect you. It's a good idea to keep a journal of your behaviours and thoughts while understanding that self-awareness is an ongoing journey.

With practice you will become more confident, efficient and grounded with an outlook that's far more positive than before. So meditate, self-reflect, acknowledge your bodily sensations, and foster an awareness of your triggers while tuning into your needs. Whether at home, at work or simply in the world, you're sure to feel better for it.

Think of a common emotion you feel that you'd like to explore more. In this diagram, write down how this emotion makes different parts of your body feel.

Five years

Twenty-five years

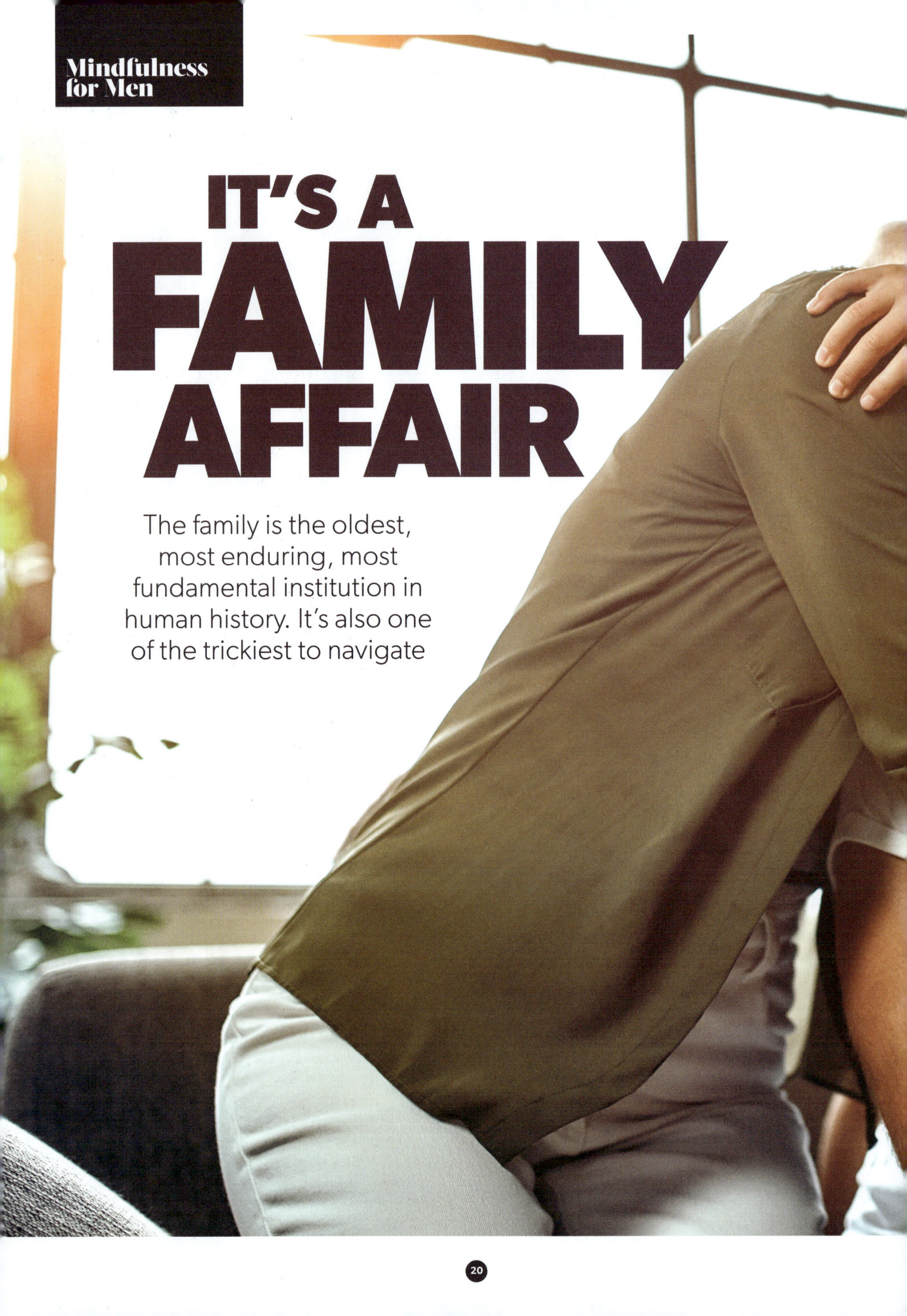

Mindfulness for Men

IT'S A FAMILY AFFAIR

The family is the oldest, most enduring, most fundamental institution in human history. It's also one of the trickiest to navigate

It's a family affair

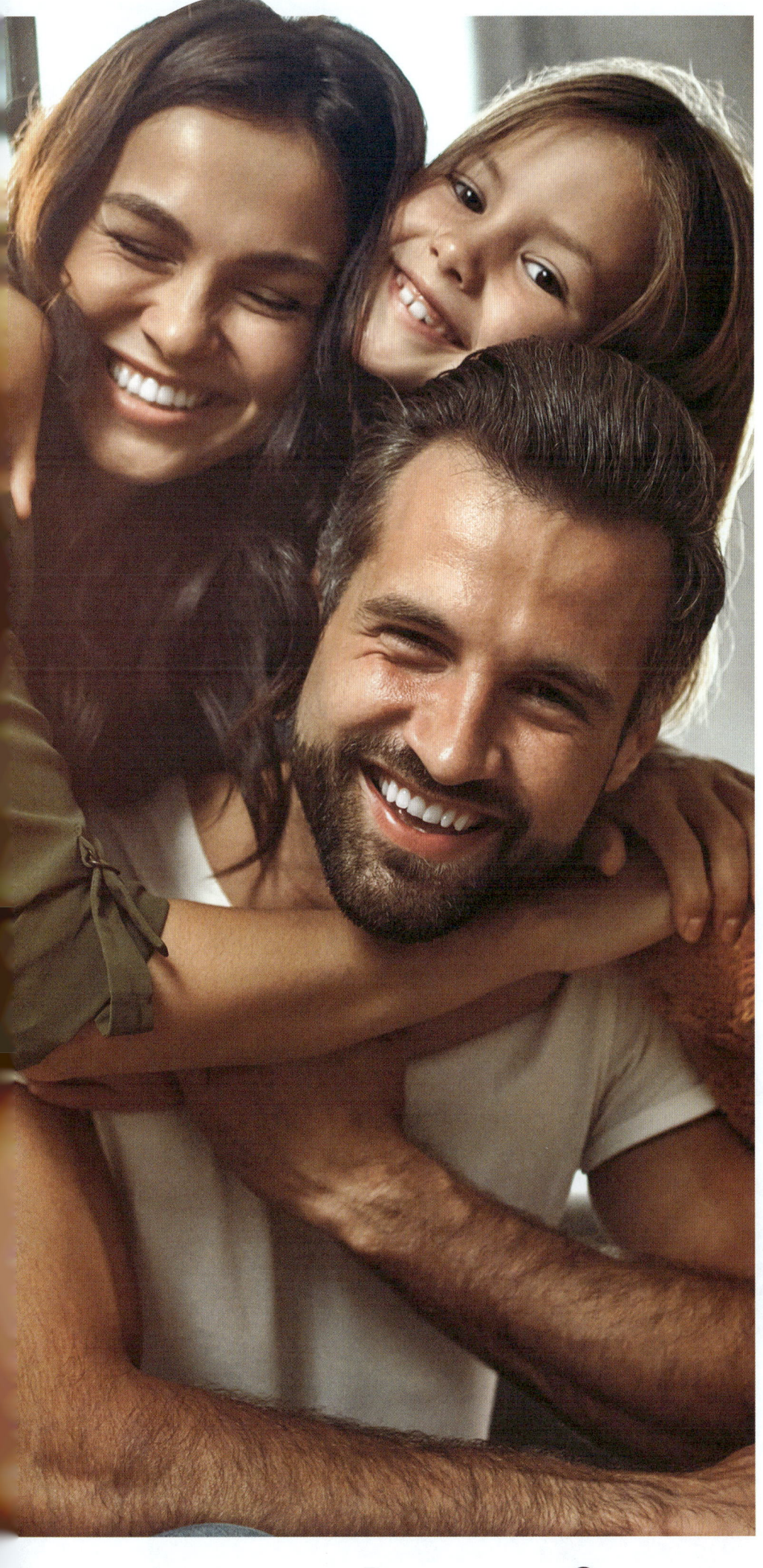

Most of us begin within a family. It might be a truncated family or one that extends through generations and innumerable relatives, but whatever its nature, a family is usually where we begin.

Famously, Tolstoy began his great novel, *Anna Karenina*, by saying, "All happy families are alike; each unhappy family is unhappy in its own way." Few quotes are better known and more spectacularly, diametrically wrong. It is happiness that is unique, finding individual expression in happy families, while it is misery that proves to be stereotypical, running through standard tropes of selfishness, repetitive behaviour patterns and immaturity. But even though it might be stereotypical, the misery produced by unhappy family relationships is all too real and extremely bitter. However, the sort of forced behaviour patterns that can lock families into their own private hells are conducive to the sort of mindful awareness that we are looking at in this book.

BEHAVIOUR PATTERNS IN FAMILIES
Families are full of roles: father, mother, daughter, son, provider, carer, student, high achiever, underachiever. We all know examples. Uncle Bill, who can fix anything. Little Jenny, the princess. Auntie Liz, who always speaks her mind. These roles are, in most cases, useful. They prevent duplication of effort – if dad is good at DIY and mum prefers cooking, then it makes sense for dad to repair the broken plug connection in the kitchen, and for mum to cook the dinner when he's done, because the various members of the family get to do what they are best at.

However, these family roles can become fixed and remarkably resistant to change, even when they have ceased to be relevant. For instance, as a child a boy might be uncoordinated and somewhat clumsy, always falling over his feet and getting his finger shut in doors. At the same time, his sister was precise and neat, quickly learning how to cook and prepare food. So after a few attempts at getting the boy to help with cooking, which ended with a mess of mangled vegetables and nearly chopping off a thumb, mum decided for the sake of everyone's health that it was best if the boy didn't do any more cooking. So the

Mindfulness for Men

son takes the family role of all-round goofball while the daughter becomes mum's little helper. That might be all very well for a while. But 20 years down the line, when the son has grown up, moved out and started a career as a chef, yet finds that his mother and sister still insist that they chop the vegetables because he can't be trusted not to cut off his own fingers, those old family roles might begin to seem a little tired. However, families can be very resistant to changing the perceived roles of their members. This is where mindfulness can prove very useful.

MINDFULNESS FOR FAMILY ROLES

As mentioned elsewhere in this book, mindfulness consists of focused attention to the present moment. It brings us into direct contact with what we are experiencing right now and, even more importantly for the functioning of family roles, it allows us to view what someone is actually doing right in front of us, and how they are doing it, rather than what they used to do ten or 20 years ago.

So suppose, growing up, your sister was a bit clumsy, full of laughter and fun but the last person to trust with giving out medicine. Now suppose 20 years have gone by and that little girl has grown up, married, and had three children, and the family has all come together for a family gathering – only to find that your sister's youngest has come down with a fever. As she goes to open the bottle of Calpol, granny, still treating your sister as her younger self, takes the bottle of Calpol from her, unscrews the child-proof lock while chuckling about how her daughter could never open these, and gives the medicine to the distressed little boy herself, while mum hovers in impotent fury.

It's under conditions of stress that families tend to fall back into their stereotyped roles, even when a moment's consideration would have shown that, having successfully raised three children, the daughter had become perfectly capable of opening a bottle of Calpol herself. At the time, it might be difficult to stop this reversion to the mean, but afterwards, should the family be willing to examine events mindfully, it would be possible for everyone to slowly come to understand how old roles had overcome present reality. To prevent their continuation, a habit of mindfulness would help prevent people slipping back into these old behavioural channels when they were no longer relevant.

Right: Practising mindfulness can make family occasions far more enjoyable

IMPERFECT IS OK
We are bombarded with images of 'perfect' families, but these are just that: images. Imperfection is not only inevitable in family life, it's healthier too.

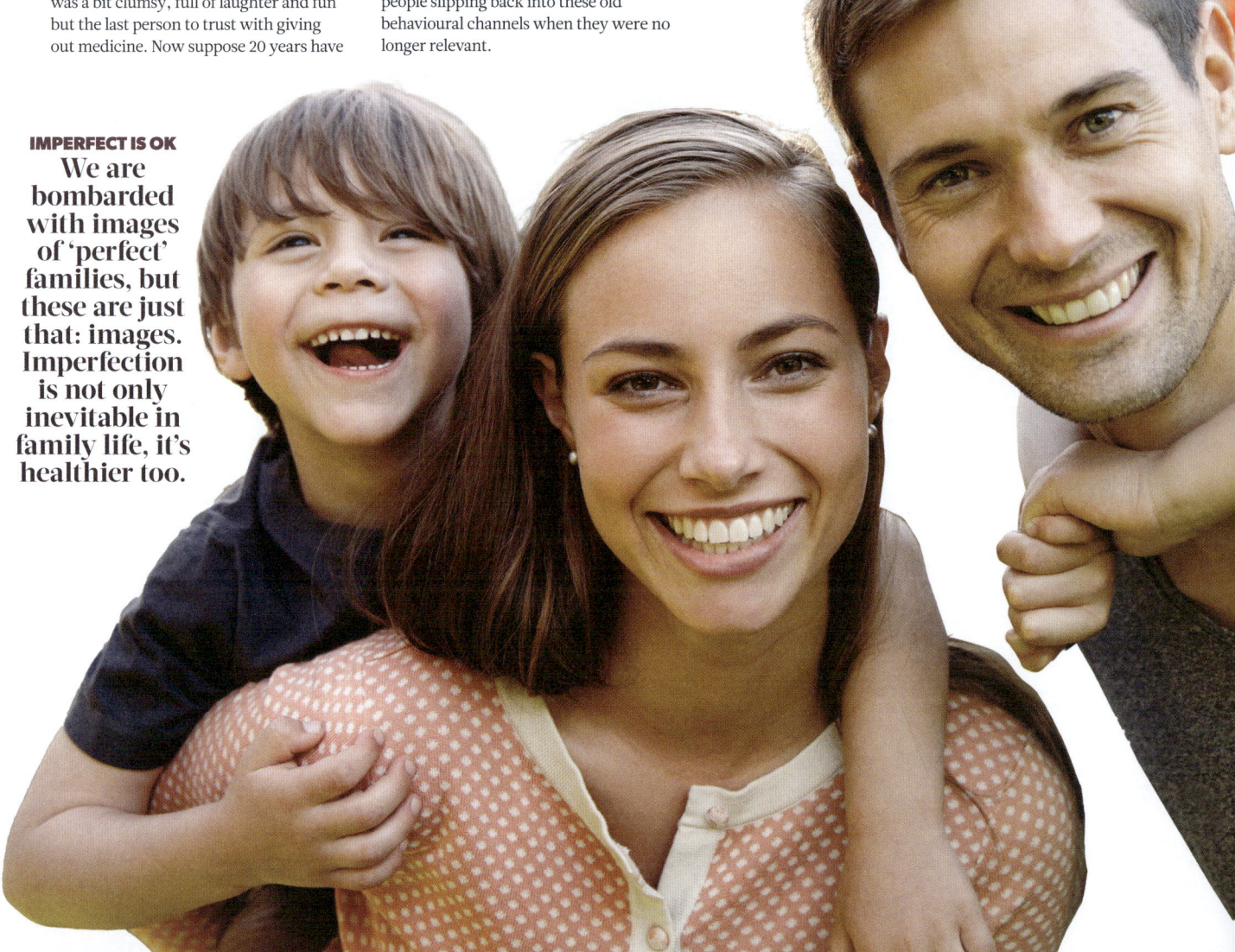

It's a family affair

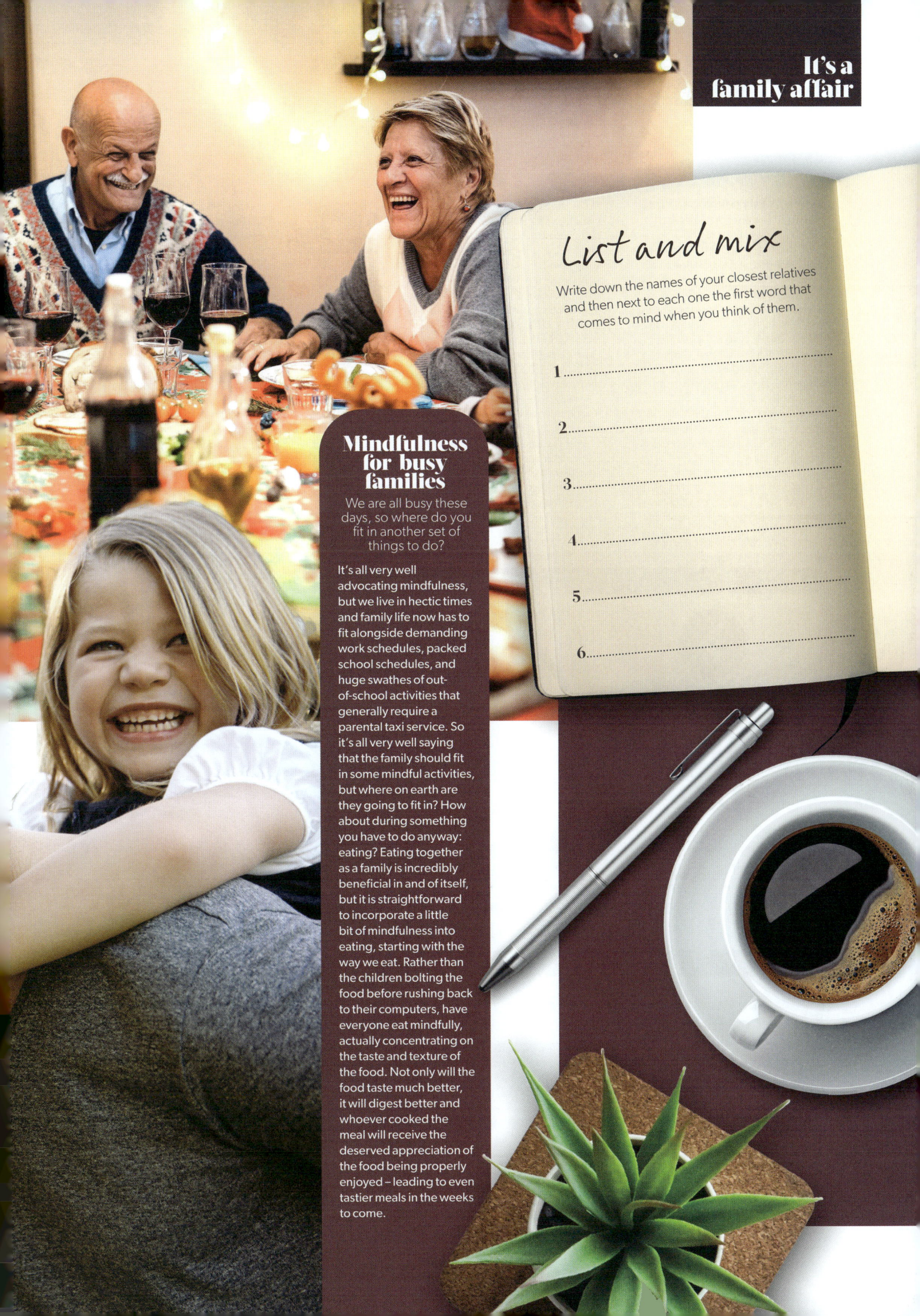

List and mix
Write down the names of your closest relatives and then next to each one the first word that comes to mind when you think of them.

1. ....
2. ....
3. ....
4. ....
5. ....
6. ....

Mindfulness for busy families
We are all busy these days, so where do you fit in another set of things to do?

It's all very well advocating mindfulness, but we live in hectic times and family life now has to fit alongside demanding work schedules, packed school schedules, and huge swathes of out-of-school activities that generally require a parental taxi service. So it's all very well saying that the family should fit in some mindful activities, but where on earth are they going to fit in? How about during something you have to do anyway: eating? Eating together as a family is incredibly beneficial in and of itself, but it is straightforward to incorporate a little bit of mindfulness into eating, starting with the way we eat. Rather than the children bolting the food before rushing back to their computers, have everyone eat mindfully, actually concentrating on the taste and texture of the food. Not only will the food taste much better, it will digest better and whoever cooked the meal will receive the deserved appreciation of the food being properly enjoyed – leading to even tastier meals in the weeks to come.

Mindfulness for Men

WHEN EVERYTHING CHANGES

You might not want or be able to have children for whatever reason. If you do decide to have a child though, it's impossible to conceive just how much of an impact they will have on your life until they arrive. If born into a family of two parents, a baby will transform a couple from a dyad into a family, and fundamentally change the existing dynamics of a relationship. Despite any intentions to the contrary, a child changes the focus of the parents. This is necessary and inevitable, but it can nevertheless come as something of a shock to one of the parents or even both parents, each being suddenly relegated from the focus of their partner's attention. Sometimes you'll feel as though you're at the bottom of a pile that includes the immediate needs of the baby and the necessity to provide for them in the future. Humanity is based upon parents sacrificing their own desires for the needs of their children – but sacrifices, by their nature, can be painful. To cope with these changes, a mindful attitude can be very helpful. Generosity is one of the key attitudes inculcated by mindfulness, an ability to entirely give of oneself to the person in front of you and to allow that person to be entirely themselves. Such an attitude is almost perfectly tuned towards coping with the inevitable stresses of adjusting to a new family life, and to bringing out the best of the child you have brought into the world.

Most parents receive their first child full of ambitions for what they will grow up to be and achieve, only to quickly learn that every child will grow into their own set of potentialities. Trying to force them into something of your own making will only stunt the child's growth, or distort it. But adopting an attitude of mindful generosity will help to bring out all the potential that is inherent in the child, as well as bring you the incalculable benefit of watching it happen.

CHILDREN WITH SPECIAL NEEDS

Over the last few decades, more children than ever before have been diagnosed with autism, ADHD, dyslexia, ADD, dyspraxia and other conditions. This has resulted in many more families needing to cope with children whose needs run beyond the usual. In these circumstances, practising mindfulness might seem difficult at best, impossible at worst. However, facing challenging situations like this mindfully may help them to have less impact on your own levels of stress. By a rigorous focus on what is in front of you at this specific moment, it becomes

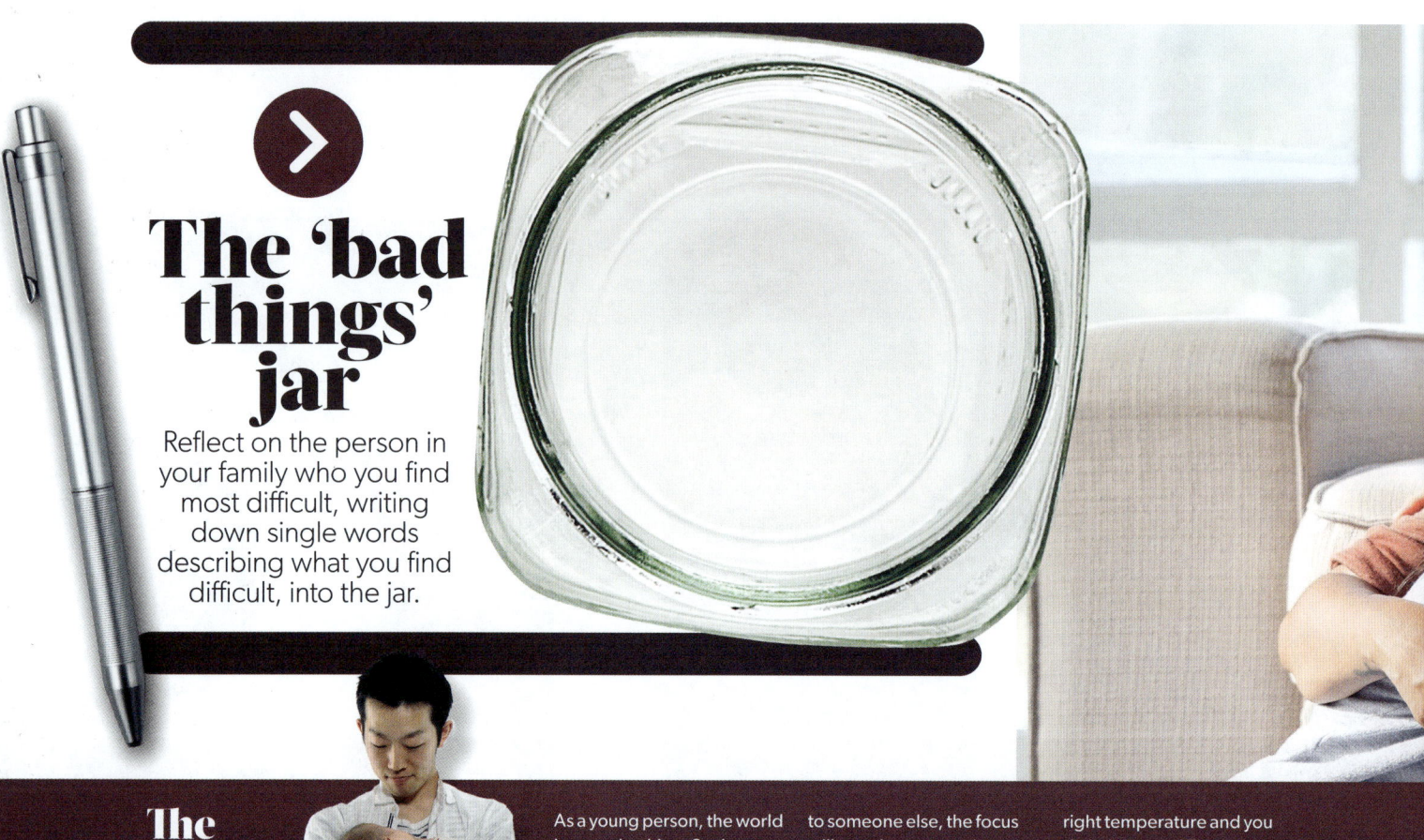

Below: Having children will change your focus and your family role

> The 'bad things' jar

Reflect on the person in your family who you find most difficult, writing down single words describing what you find difficult, into the jar.

The needs of others

Why suddenly finding out that you're really not the most important person in the world is actually a liberation

As a young person, the world is your plaything. Society – or at least advertisers – holds up the achievements of your ambitions, your wishes and your desires as the very definition of purpose in life. It's all about you. Even when you find and commit to someone else, the focus still remains on you: the way they make you feel, the way you hunger for each other. But when a baby comes along, everything changes. The person who doted on you is suddenly demanding that you get that bottle the right temperature and you do it right now! The baby's hungry. From top of the pile, you might find yourself at the bottom of the family heap: the person whose wishes, needs and desires are now least important. But you know what? Embrace that. Look

possible to see better what is actually there, hopefully allowing for a better understanding of the reasons for the particular behaviour, as well as making it possible to deal with this incident on its own, rather than subsuming it under the mantle of all the previous incidents that you have endured. Dealing with it fresh allows for fresh approaches, as well as helping you to assess accurately whether there was anything you could have done to stop it.

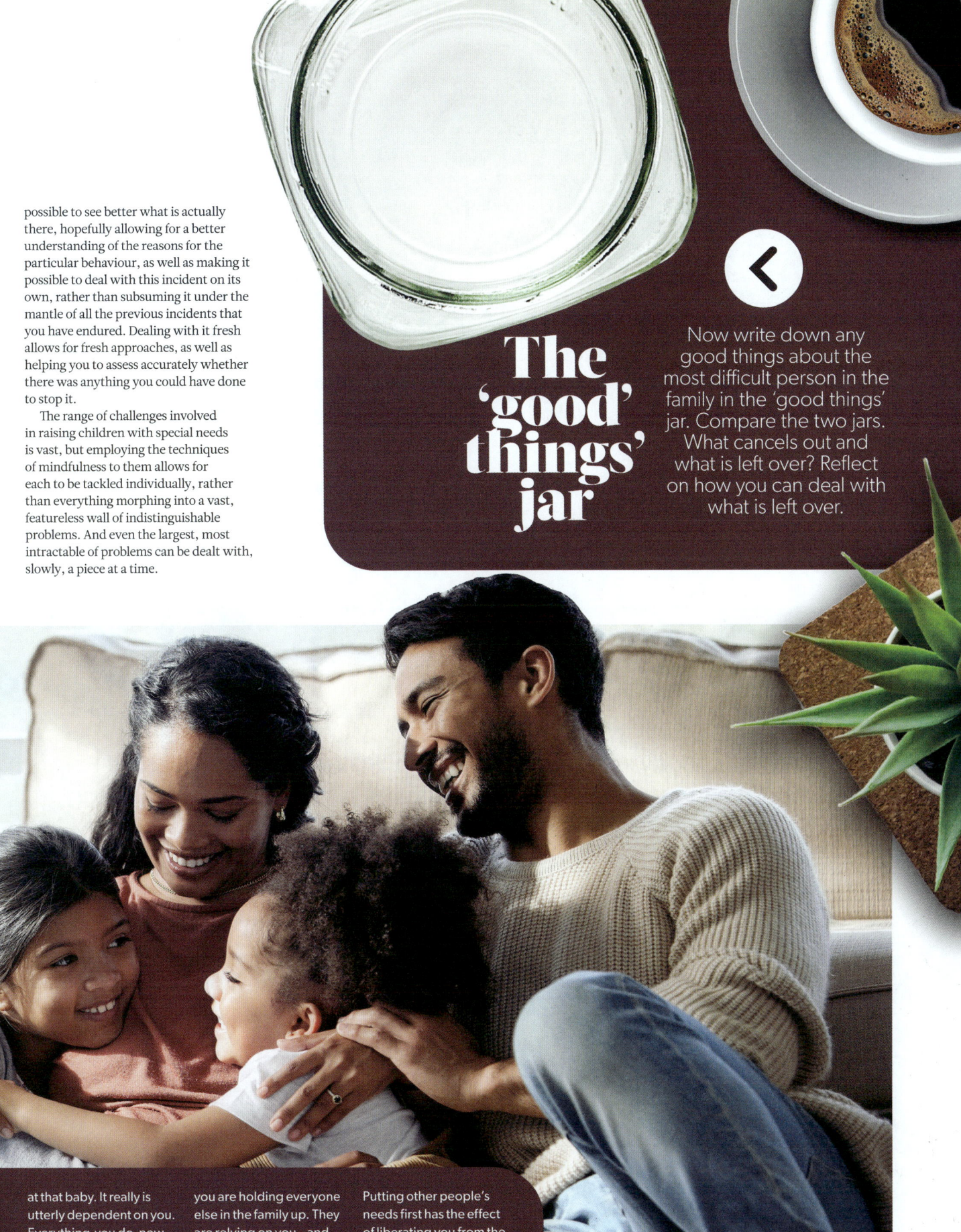

The range of challenges involved in raising children with special needs is vast, but employing the techniques of mindfulness to them allows for each to be tackled individually, rather than everything morphing into a vast, featureless wall of indistinguishable problems. And even the largest, most intractable of problems can be dealt with, slowly, a piece at a time.

The 'good' things' jar

Now write down any good things about the most difficult person in the family in the 'good things' jar. Compare the two jars. What cancels out and what is left over? Reflect on how you can deal with what is left over.

at that baby. It really is utterly dependent on you. Everything you do, now, matters, really matters in a way that mastering the newest computer game never really did. Yes, you are the bottom of the heap but that might be because you are holding everyone else in the family up. They are relying on you – and they can do so because they know that you are putting them before your own desires. For a new father, this comes as an extraordinary revelation. Putting other people's needs first has the effect of liberating you from the idols of contemporary culture while putting you in contact with the oldest, deepest stream in human history: looking after and raising your children.

Mindfulness for Men

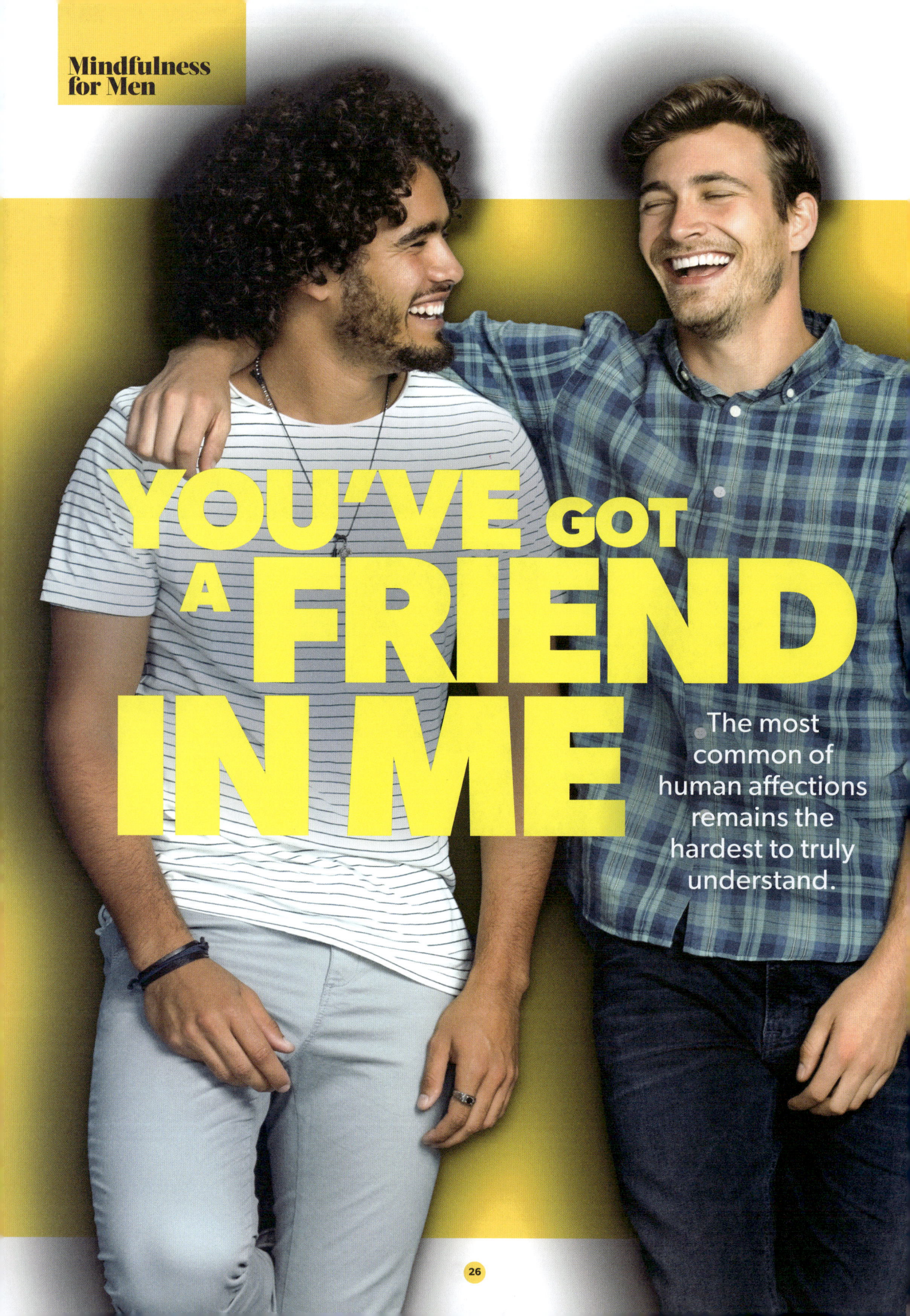

YOU'VE GOT A FRIEND IN ME

The most common of human affections remains the hardest to truly understand.

You've got a friend in me

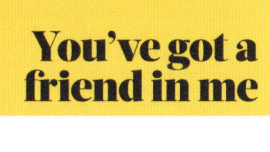

Good friend/bad friend
If there's a friend whose influence you are uncertain about, reflect on your reactions the last time you saw them and write them down here.

AIM HIGH
Set a shared goal with your friend or friends and work to achieve it.

T he ancient Greeks, who had a passion for naming things, did so with love too. Where we are stuck with just the one word, the Greeks assigned four different words for four different types of love: the love of parents for children (storge), romantic love (eros), unconditional love (agape) and the love between friends (philia). This philia, the affection uniting friends, the ancients regarded as the highest and purest form of love, since it was unselfish and disinterested.

The writer CS Lewis examined these four different types of love in his book *The Four Loves*, which remains the most valuable treatment of friendship written in the last century, and pointed out that where the other three forms of love are exclusive, binding people together in a way that necessarily excludes others (if you fall in love with someone you're not going to be making puppy eyes at another person), philia, the love of friends, is intrinsically inclusive because it is based, fundamentally, on a shared appreciation of something. Two lovers stand face to face, staring at each other, two friends stand side by side, engaged with what they enjoy in common. As Lewis wrote, 'The typical expression of opening Friendship would be something like, "What? You too? I thought I was the only one".'

TRUE FRIENDSHIP
Being based on a common interest or passion, friendship is broadened and deepened by finding others who share the same interest. For many, this is the fundamental nature of friendship, a nature that often develops into the creation of societies of shared interests. There have been many failed attempts to re-engage older, lonely men with society. In particular, widowers find it very difficult, and well-meaning efforts telling them to express their feelings of loss are commonly met with complete failure. What does work is finding a group of men with a shared interest. As a locus of activity and shared worth, you would be hard put to beat the effort that goes into your local model railway society: not only are the layouts extraordinary pieces of engineering but the society of like-minded individuals gives lonely men a path back into society without the focus being them and their feelings. Talking about themselves and opening up about their feelings will often then follow naturally and comfortably.

Because true friendship is based upon a shared interest and passion, it is, by its very definition, mindful. Being engaged in a common pursuit, be that hiking, the theatre or the gym, often involves concentrating on it together, being mindful without even realising that that is what you're doing.

THE IMPORTANCE OF GOOD FRIENDS
Because friendship is so often group based, people have sometimes used it in an effort to redeem those who are having difficulties. For instance, suppose

Finding friends

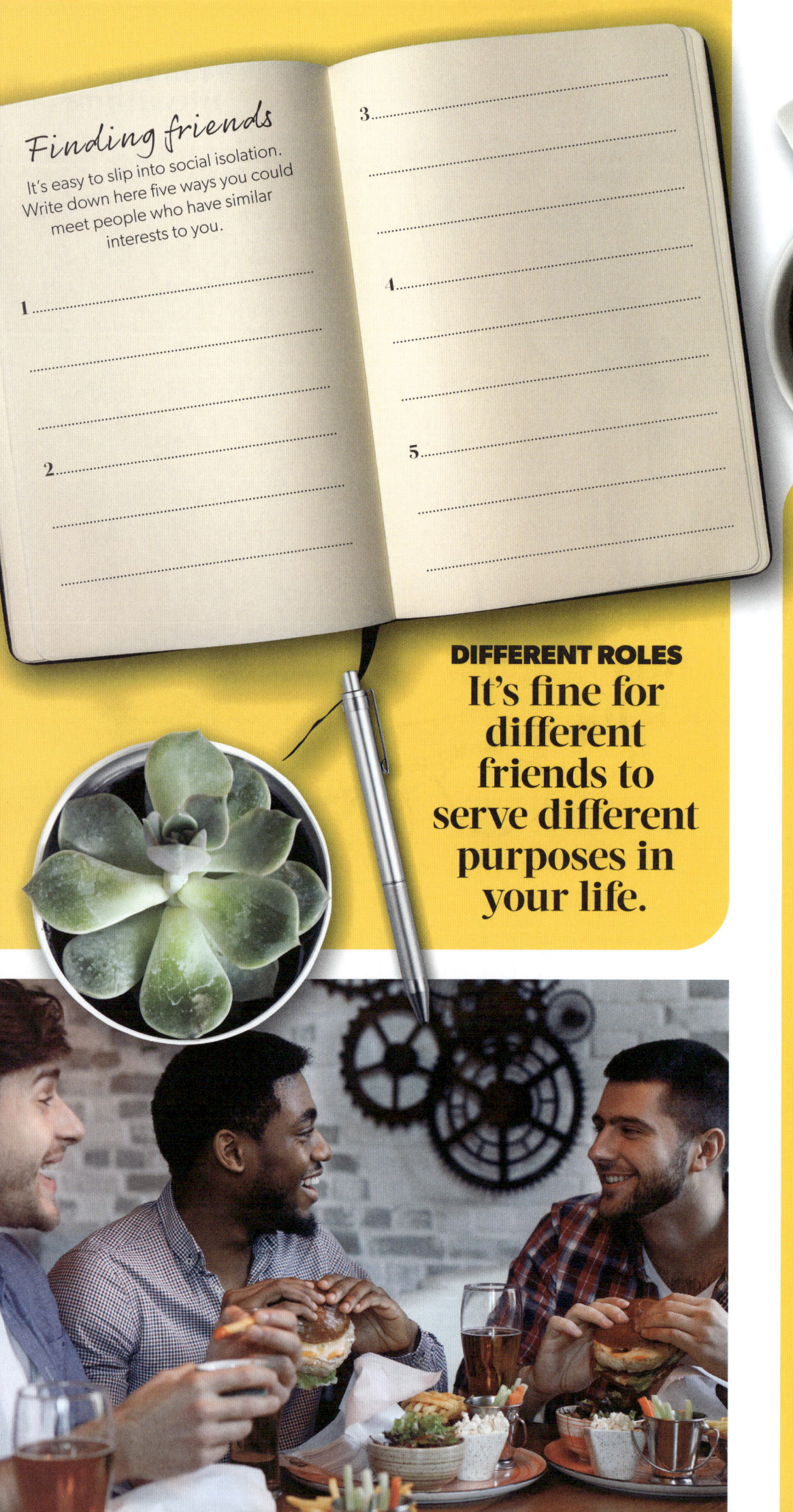

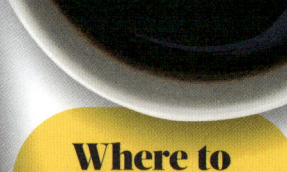

It's easy to slip into social isolation. Write down here five ways you could meet people who have similar interests to you.

1. ....
....
....

2. ....
....
....

3. ....
....
....

4. ....
....

5. ....
....

DIFFERENT ROLES
It's fine for different friends to serve different purposes in your life.

Where to make friends
A lot of us find it difficult to make friends, particularly as we age

Throughout our lives, friendships present a whole host of challenges. As children, we face playground squabbles, but are protected by our teachers, family, and lack of inhibitions. As we navigate adolescence, friendships might become more intense, but are arguably one of the most important aspects of our lives. And as we enter adulthood, cultivating friendships becomes harder still, as a self-consciousness takes over. Inhibitions and life experiences often make it harder to make friends as we get older – perhaps we've been let down by so-called good friends; maybe our friends have changed or their lives have progressed at a different rate to our own; or perhaps we become lazy and stop making an effort with people. It's easy to fall out of contact and end up feeling lonely. Human connections are vital for our mental wellbeing, though, and nurturing friendships should be a priority. This is most easily done by associations of common interests. The shared interests, and the implied shared values that go with those interests, will help to facilitate friendships to ensure that we don't end up lonely and unfulfilled.

You've got a friend in me

you're a manager at a big corporation and you have one brilliant team who work together and achieve stellar results, but you're also responsible for a single, clever but troubled individual who finds it difficult to work with other people. The temptation would obviously be to put this person in with the top team: their proven cohesion will surely accommodate this individual's difficulties, rather like an oyster turns a piece of grit into a pearl.

Unfortunately, that's often not how it works. Research suggests that rather than the good group lifting up the bad individual, the bad apple will drag down the group, fracturing its previous cohesiveness and turning its members against each other. Similarly, among a group of friends, a single bitter member of the group can curdle everything.

CHOOSE GOOD FRIENDS
Friendship is important at any age, but assumes a paramount importance in early life, particularly between the late teens and late twenties. This is when friendship is most important and formative. When it works, it can transform a bunch of youngsters into something special: The Beatles were fast friends whose friendship fostered music that changed the world. But while good friends can produce extraordinary results, bad friends can lead us down into the abyss.

This is where mindful attention to a friendship can be vital. Suppose you have an old, dear friend. They've been around for years and while they might have gone a little off the rails recently, they're still your friend. You still hang out with them. But pay attention to the effects of being with this friend. Do you find that you are energised and alert? Or do the demons that are affecting them start affecting you too when you are together? Do you feel better for having seen them, or worse? Too many promising lives have spiralled downwards as a result of holding on to a friendship that has ceased to be a true friendship but has rather become a device for an individual set on self destruction to have company on the way down.

A good friend is one who wants what is good for you. Being with a true friend makes you a better person and makes them a better person. If the opposite happens, and they are dragging you down, then it's time to let go.

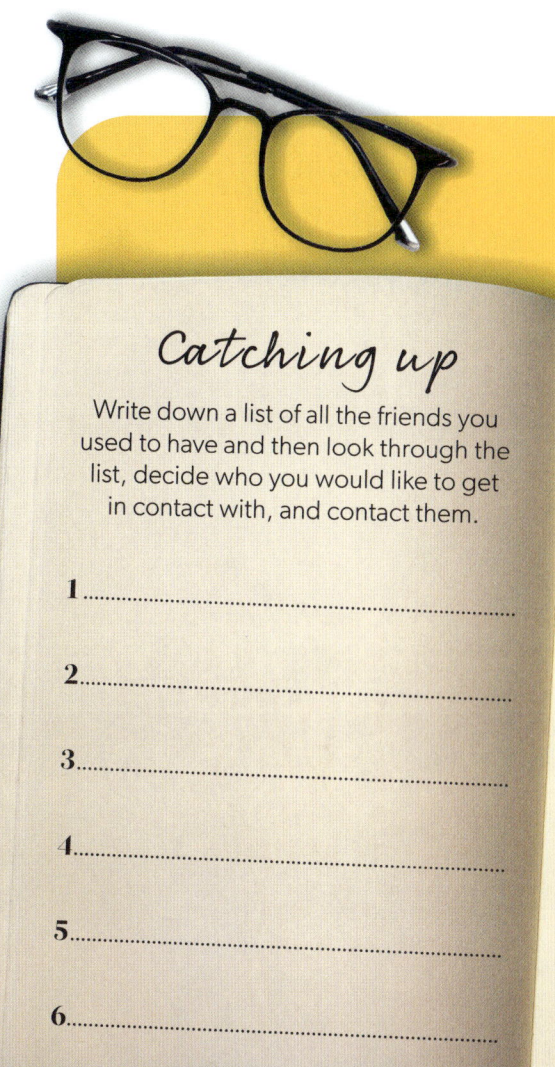

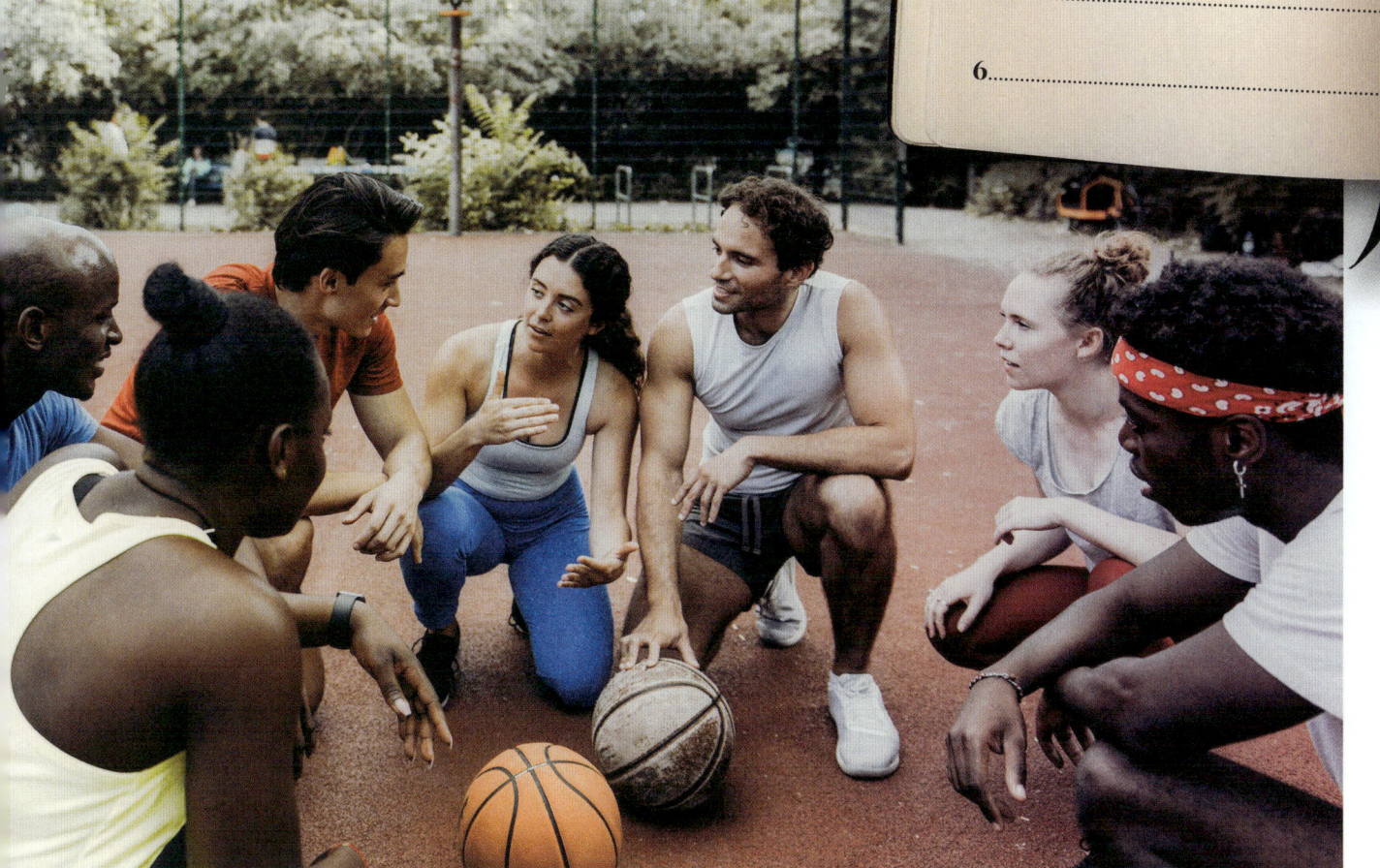

Catching up

Write down a list of all the friends you used to have and then look through the list, decide who you would like to get in contact with, and contact them.

1..
2..
3..
4..
5..
6..

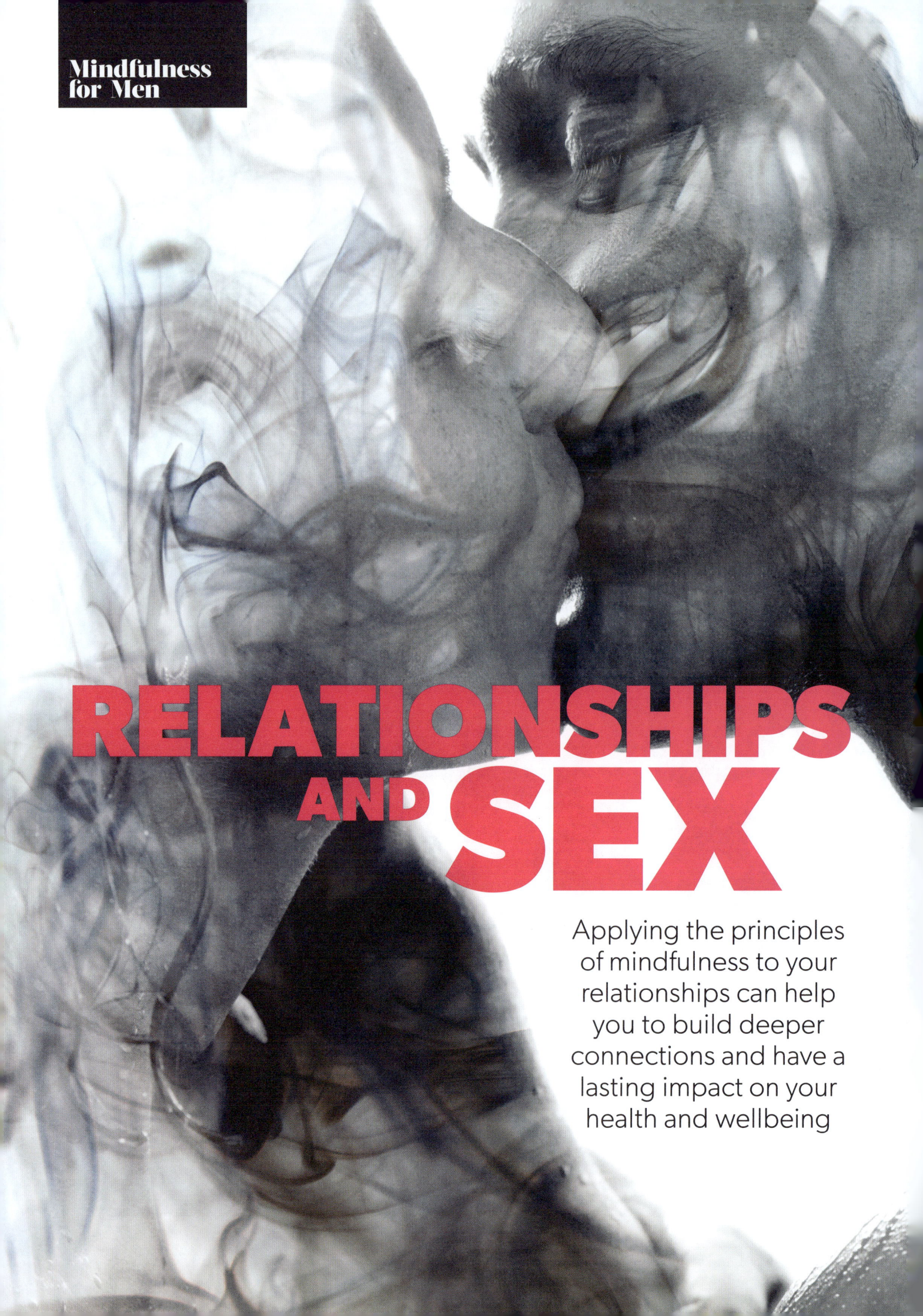

Mindfulness for Men

RELATIONSHIPS AND SEX

Applying the principles of mindfulness to your relationships can help you to build deeper connections and have a lasting impact on your health and wellbeing

Relationships and sex

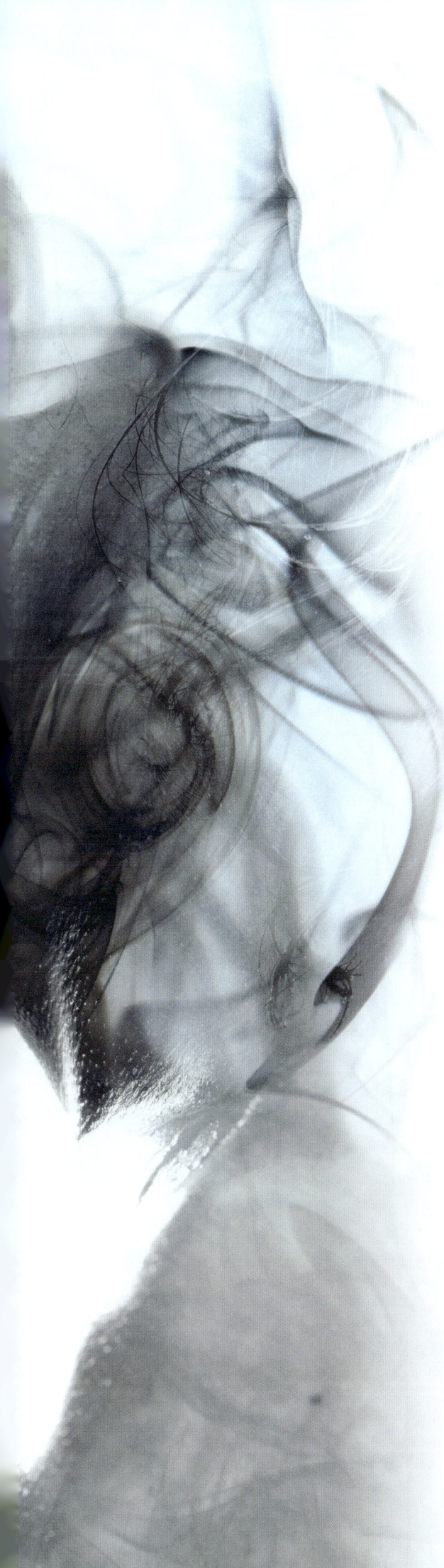

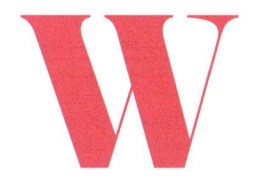

Whether you currently have a partner or not, being mindful about the kind of relationship you want in your life is important. Mindfulness relies on a conscious awareness about all aspects of our lives. In terms of a relationship, it means being aware of your partner and their feelings, being honest about your own thoughts and feelings, and being true to what you want out of your relationship. If you're not in a relationship, then it's about being mindful of whether you do want a partner or not, what kind of relationship you're looking for, and what barriers might be holding you back.

MINDFULNESS IN LONG-TERM RELATIONSHIPS

In a long-term relationship or marriage, it can be easy to fall into a comfortable rhythm and routine over time. We form habits when we're around the same person a lot of the time. This can create a feeling of security and support for some; others might find routine too restrictive and lacking in spontaneity. There is no right or wrong way for a long-term relationship to unfold, but it's important to retain openness and honesty.

This is where mindfulness comes in. Being mindful in a relationship means spending some time exploring your own feelings around your relationships. Are you happy? What is good about your partnership? What do you feel is holding your relationship back? Only you can answer these questions. It's also about being mindful of your partner and the way they are feeling. It's important to take the time to talk, to be honest, to ask questions, and to truly listen to the answers that your partner gives, being open to whatever they have to say. Many of us can find this process of communication hard, even with someone we love. It can make us feel vulnerable and unsure, but having the chance to be honest and open with each other will help to strengthen bonds and build trust.

Your relationship will change over the months and years. There will always be periods of time when you feel happier in your relationship than other times. This is a normal ebb and flow. Relationships can be impacted by changes in your life, such as having children, needing to care for an elderly parent, moving house, switching career or getting a promotion, grief and so on, and without addressing these changes, relationships can suffer under stress.

By taking a regular audit of your relationship, you can identify any issues or problems sooner, before they have a chance to develop and grow. Try to make regular space to spend time together and just talk, listening honestly to each other and addressing any new changes. Be patient with each other; sometimes change happens to only one partner and they may have things they need to work through on their own. Be mindful as to when you need to be there to comfort and listen, and when you need to step back and create space. Mindfulness in this way can help you to practise compassion and develop a deeper understanding within your relationship.

LOSS OF A RELATIONSHIP

Sometimes relationships will come to an end, and there are many reasons why this might happen. This can be a difficult situation to navigate, and it comes with a lot of feelings that can be overwhelming.

If you ended the relationship, take some time to think over your decision. Why did you end the relationship? Was there anything that could have been done to take things down a different path? If you're sure it was the right decision, consider those factors and think of how these may impact on any future relationships. If your relationship was ended by your partner, then you may feel hurt, angry or regretful. Don't be afraid of these feelings; it's only natural to question whether you did something wrong, whether you could have acted in a different way, or to feel confused by your partner's reasons. Accept that you can't always know the answers, but be kind to yourself – you are not responsible for someone else's actions.

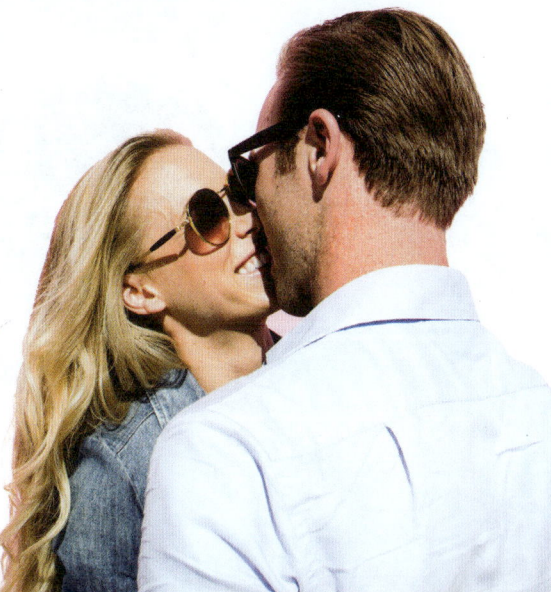

> **DIARISE A DATE NIGHT**
> Be aware of when life is taking over, and book in a date night with your partner to reconnect and talk.

Mindfulness for Men

However the relationship ended, give yourself the time you need to heal. This can be harder when there is a divorce to navigate, a shared home, children, pets or joint possessions. There will be a period of time when the practicalities need to be discussed and dealt with. Be kind to yourself during this time, and make sure that you practise self-care. Talk to friends and family about the way you are feeling; you don't have to navigate these big life changes on your own. It's also good to reflect on your relationship. It might give you clarity over what you are looking for from future partners, or even whether you want a future partner – you may make the decision that you need to be on your own for a while.

Bereavement is a painful situation to navigate; the death of a partner is complex and the feelings associated with this can be overwhelming. It's worth seeking professional help if you can, through a therapist or support service, to help deal with the complex emotions that surround grief. Practising mindfulness and introducing meditation may help support your wellbeing during this difficult time.

Below: Being open and honest with your partner helps to strengthen bonds and build trust in your relationship

SEEKING A RELATIONSHIP

If you're not in a relationship, you can still be mindful about the prospect of one. Consider whether you're happy not being in a relationship – many people enjoy being on their own and like their own company. You might feel like you want an intimate connection with another person or people, but don't want a full-time relationship. Or maybe you are in a place where you do want to seek a partner for a more committed relationship. Be honest about where you are in your life right now and what you want from your relationships. Don't feel you have to be

5-senses exercise
During intimacy, note down here…

5 THINGS YOU CAN SEE
1 ....
2 ....
3 ....
4 ....
5 ....

4 THINGS YOU CAN FEEL
1 ....
2 ....
3 ....
4 ....

3 THINGS YOU CAN HEAR
1 ....
2 ....
3 ....

2 THINGS YOU CAN SMELL
1 ....
2 ....

1 THING YOU CAN TASTE
1 ....

5 mindful relationship tips
Try to incorporate these tips into your relationship to build connection and intimacy

1 SHOW GRATITUDE
Tell your partner why you feel grateful for them and when you appreciate something they do for you. It doesn't always have to be the big things.

2 DIGITAL DETOX
Set aside a regular time every week where you and your partner put away your phones and tablets, turn off the TV, and spend some time together without any distractions.

Show you care

Write down a list of things to do to show your partner that you appreciate them, and then work out a schedule to actually do them.

....
....
....
....
....
....
....

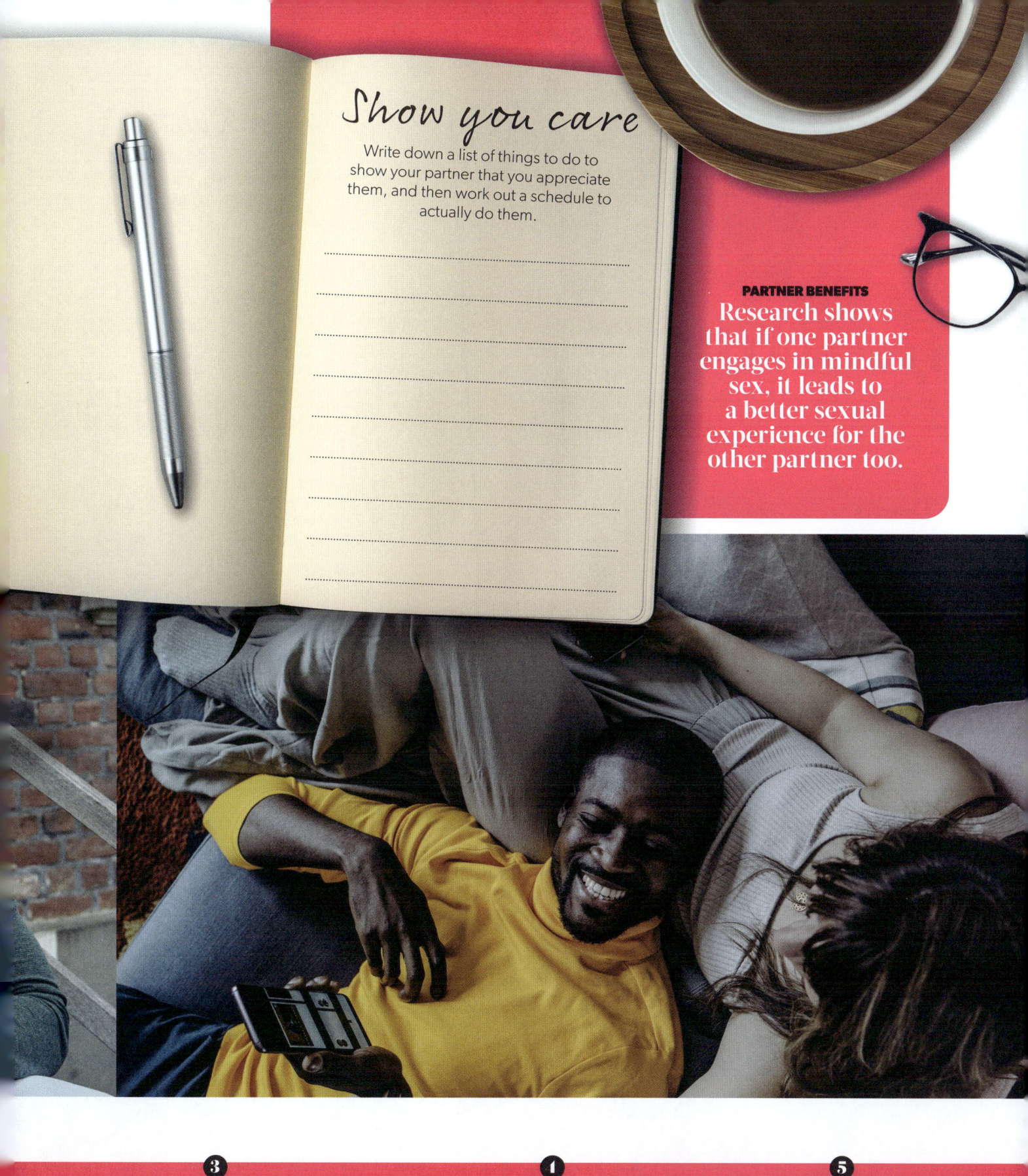

PARTNER BENEFITS
Research shows that if one partner engages in mindful sex, it leads to a better sexual experience for the other partner too.

3
ASK QUESTIONS
You might feel like you know your partner inside out, but there is always the opportunity to learn more about each other. Ask them how their day went, if they're worried about anything or if they need to talk. Or just ask lighter questions, such as their favourite time of day, or where they'd love to go on holiday.

4
SPEND TIME APART
It's really important in relationships to spend time doing things individually as well as together. There will be hobbies and interests that you enjoy that your partner doesn't. It's good for your wellbeing to do these hobbies and spend time with other people. And make sure that your partner has time to do the things that they enjoy too. It will help you both to feel more fulfilled and happier.

5
TRY SOMETHING NEW TOGETHER
Doing new things takes us out of our comfort zone. By doing something new with a partner, you will have a shared experience and you can support each other, as well as have something fresh to talk about and bond over.

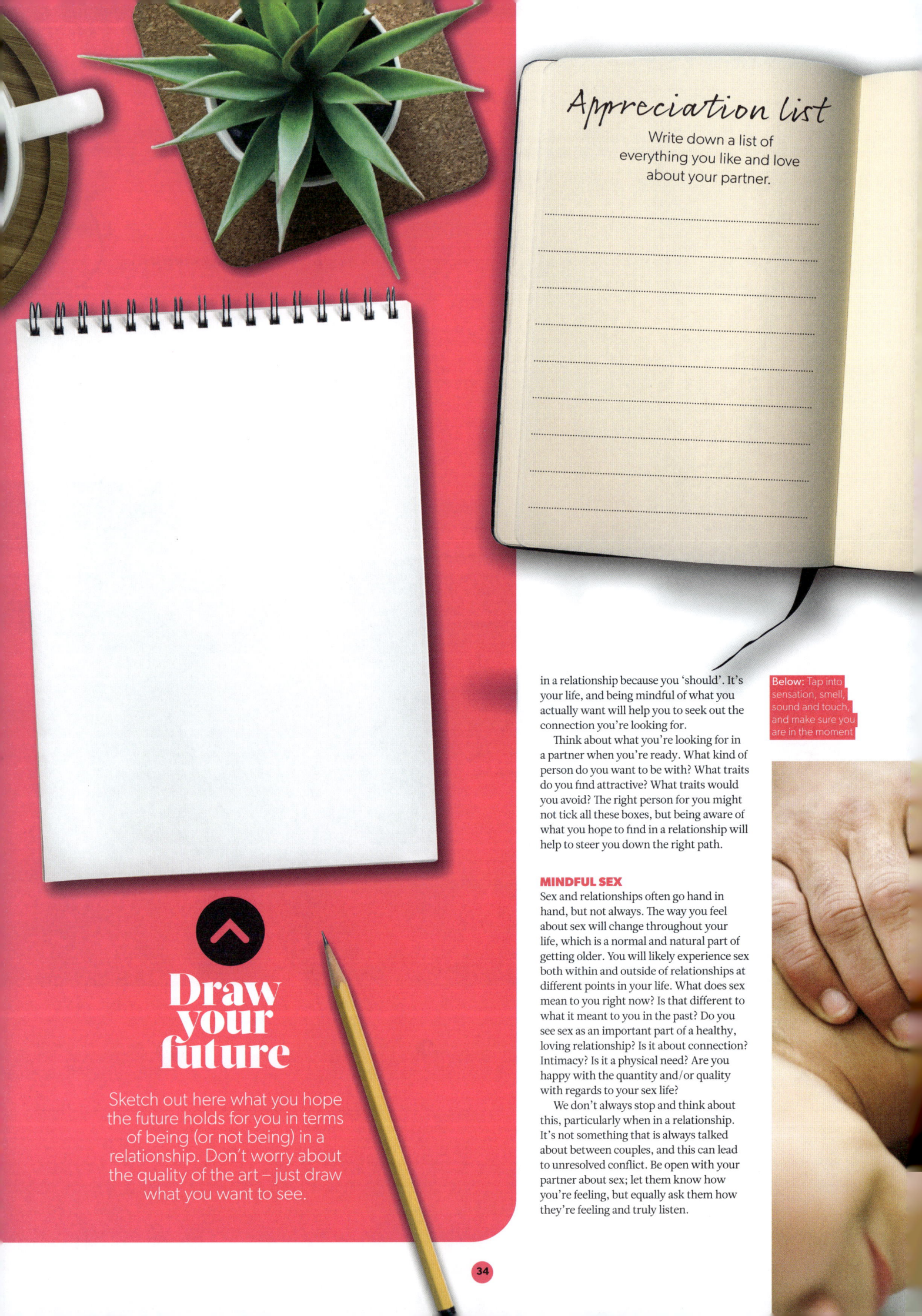

Appreciation list
Write down a list of everything you like and love about your partner.

Draw your future
Sketch out here what you hope the future holds for you in terms of being (or not being) in a relationship. Don't worry about the quality of the art – just draw what you want to see.

in a relationship because you 'should'. It's your life, and being mindful of what you actually want will help you to seek out the connection you're looking for.

Think about what you're looking for in a partner when you're ready. What kind of person do you want to be with? What traits do you find attractive? What traits would you avoid? The right person for you might not tick all these boxes, but being aware of what you hope to find in a relationship will help to steer you down the right path.

MINDFUL SEX
Sex and relationships often go hand in hand, but not always. The way you feel about sex will change throughout your life, which is a normal and natural part of getting older. You will likely experience sex both within and outside of relationships at different points in your life. What does sex mean to you right now? Is that different to what it meant to you in the past? Do you see sex as an important part of a healthy, loving relationship? Is it about connection? Intimacy? Is it a physical need? Are you happy with the quantity and/or quality with regards to your sex life?

We don't always stop and think about this, particularly when in a relationship. It's not something that is always talked about between couples, and this can lead to unresolved conflict. Be open with your partner about sex; let them know how you're feeling, but equally ask them how they're feeling and truly listen.

Below: Tap into sensation, smell, sound and touch, and make sure you are in the moment

Relationships and sex

Mindful sex
Being in the present moment can help make sex great again

It's perhaps not entirely surprising that being intensely in the present moment and completely aware of physical sensations can serve to make sex more intense, more pleasurable and more fulfilling. What is perhaps more surprising is that it's taken so long for this attitude to sex to be appreciated for its utility. In fact, a technique that is, to all intents and purposes, identical to mindful sex has been used by sex therapists since the pioneering work of Masters and Johnson in the 1950s, when they encouraged clients to focus on their sensations rather than obsessing upon the goal of achieving an orgasm. The simple fact is that anxiety, and its complement, distraction, are inimical to good sex. For men, the primary drivers of sexual anxiety are erectile dysfunction and premature ejaculation. In both cases, the anxiety provoked by the fear of not being able to perform properly in bed leads to exactly the outcome that is feared. By removing the focus from the fear and concentrating on the present moment, with all its amazing array of sensations and emotions, is to defuse the anxiety and the focus on what will happen to concentrating on what is happening. This shift of focus allows for the gradual reworking of attitudes and aims with respect to sex: with work, it becomes an act of mutual pleasure-giving rather than a performance upon which you are judged or on which you judge yourself.

Whether you're in a relationship or not, there are benefits of being mindful about sex. In a broader sense, knowing what sex means to you will help you to engage in it more authentically and be aware of what you desire. Learn what you like and don't like by tuning into your body and the way you feel – you will get more out of your sexual relationships.

But there is also mindfulness around the act of sex itself. It's all too easy to let life intrude into the bedroom, bringing stress and worry in with you, not to mention digital devices that beep and buzz with notifications. Make a commitment to leave all of that outside the door. Focus on your partner, and bring awareness to the way you are feeling. Tap into sensation, smell, sound, touch… and most importantly, be in the moment. If thoughts try to intrude, gently push them away and bring your mind back to the present moment.

Sex and relationships can be impacted by other things that are happening in our lives. If we're stressed or worried, experiencing a mental illness, working too hard, not taking time for hobbies and so on, then our relationships and our attitude towards sex will begin to suffer as a result. When you take the time to look out for yourself, and be mindful around exercise, diet, self-care, sleep and how you spend your downtime, you will feel happier, calmer and more focused – all of which will feed into your relationships and have a positive impact.

PRACTISE GRATITUDE
Being grateful can change a disappointment into a deep encounter with the true soul of someone else. Gratitude brings joy. Embrace it.

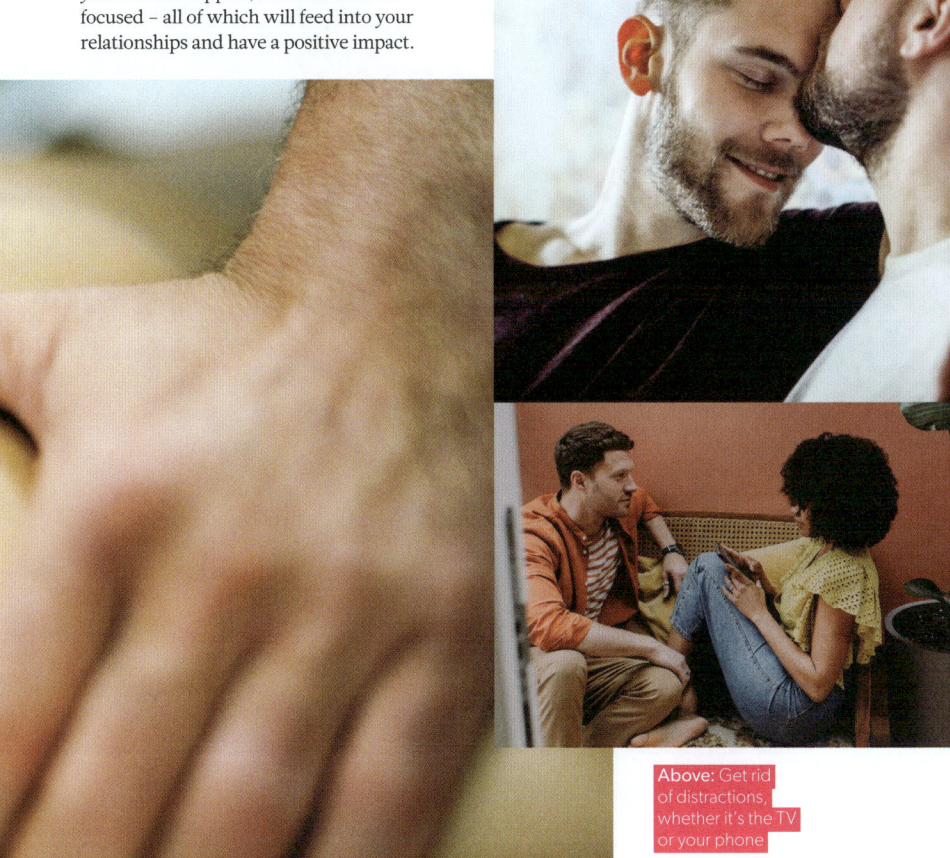

Above: Get rid of distractions, whether it's the TV or your phone

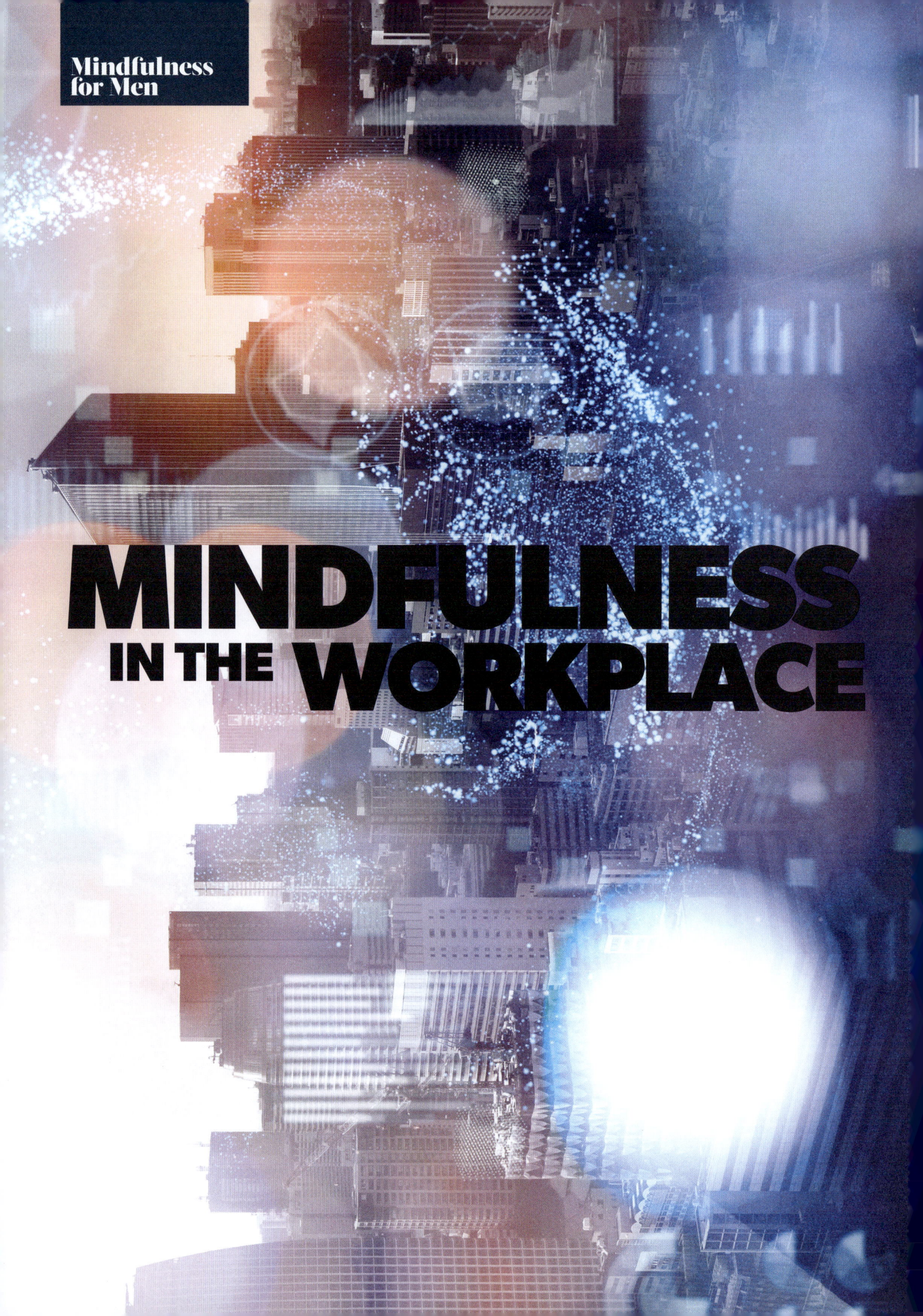

Mindfulness for Men

MINDFULNESS
IN THE WORKPLACE

Mindfulness in the workplace

How a close focus on the present moment can turbo-charge the rest of your career

O n the face of it, mindfulness does not seem to have a lot to do with jobs and careers. After all, its public image suggests sitting cross-legged, with eyes closed, while breathing slowly and evenly, and all the while becoming more and more aware that you really have to sneeze.

Aitchoo!

So, on the face of it, not a practice designed to turbocharge a career or to help select one among the many different paths we can take, jobs-wise, today. In a book concentrating on mindfulness for men, another concern is that mindfulness classes have a strong tendency to be heavily skewed towards women. A 2019 study in the *Journal of Women's Health* showed that just over 10% of the women surveyed had practised some form of meditation in the previous year compared to just over 5% of men[1]. In part, this is because meditation practices are naturally perceived to involve a degree of introspection, which some men find uncomfortable, but even more so because these practices are often advertised as being excellent ways of coming to terms with, and understanding, the emotions.

There seems to be a cross-cultural trend that men are less inclined to express emotions than women. It does not necessarily mean that men feel less or have fewer emotions, but most cultures socialise the expression of emotions by men and women differently. While this is something that needs to change, and gradually is changing in much of the Western world, marketing mindfulness as a tool towards getting in contact with one's emotions while in company with a group of other people will often make it less appealing to many men.

However, many studies have shown that mindfulness meditation can be very helpful, both in pursuing a career and even in deciding what career to follow in the first place. If you're keen to explore this further but feel hesitant or out of your comfort zone, a focus on its positive outcomes, as well as options to pursue the practice in private, might help you to get started.

1. www.ncbi.nlm.nih.gov/pmc/articles/PMC6909713

Mindfulness for Men

Living the dream?

List the top three jobs and/or careers you wanted to do as a child.
Do you wish you were doing one of these rather than your current job?

1 ....
  ....

2 ....
  ....

3 ....
  ....

5 questions about your current job

DOES IT UTILISE YOUR TALENTS?
....
....

DO YOU OFTEN LOSE YOURSELF IN YOUR WORK?
....

DO YOU HAVE A CLEAR CAREER GOAL?
....
....

DOES YOUR WORK MAKE YOU EXCITED?
....
....

IS YOUR WORK ENVIRONMENT SUPPORTIVE?
....

HAVE A GROWTH MINDSET
Be open to new possibilities, so that even negative feedback can be seen as an opportunity to improve.

HOW IS MINDFULNESS RELEVANT TO MY CAREER?

In its simplest form, mindfulness is paying attention. It's living in the moment. It's focus. It's concentration. It's many of the things that anyone trying to get on with their career would find useful. At a more formal level, mindfulness is difficult to define precisely, but researchers agree that it is the consciousness focused in the present, with the practitioner paying particular attention to internal and external stimuli. An important aspect of mindfulness is that the practitioner does not evaluate any of his thoughts, feelings, ideas or reactions: they simply experience them in an open and accepting manner.

As such, mindfulness works before the higher concepts with which we usually engage with the world and other people, such as deciding, 'That's stupid', or 'She's upset'. By paying mindful attention, you aim to see the world as it presents itself to you in the moment, without your normal filters – 'He wants my job, that's why he's suggesting we change the report' – in place. By seeing the suggested change in itself, without reference to any rivalry with a colleague, we may realise that it presents a significant improvement, and adopting it would not, in fact, be a sign of weakness but one of strength.

MINDFULNESS IN THE WORKPLACE

Given that many men prefer results-based reasons for adopting a practice that is outside their comfort zone, here are some of the findings from researchers as to the positive benefits of practising mindfulness at work:

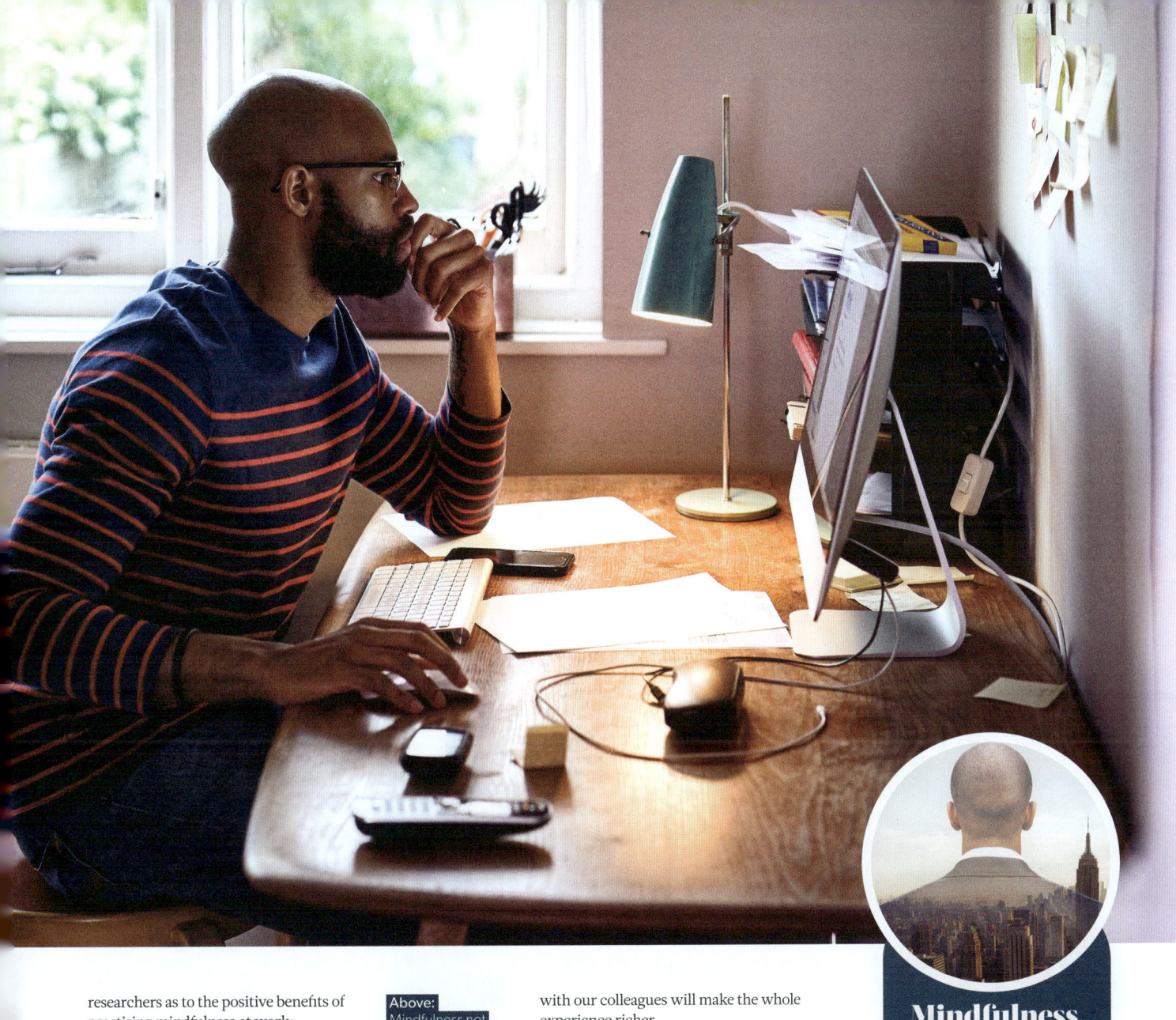

- **GREATER FLEXIBILITY OF RESPONSE**
- **HIGHER LEVELS OF PERSISTENCE AND SELF-DETERMINATION IN TASKS**
- **LESS PROCRASTINATION**
- **GREATER RESILIENCE**
- **BETTER MEMORY**
- **BETTER INTUITION**

And, what's more, workers who practise mindfulness generally report that they enjoy their jobs more than before. A large factor in improving work appreciation is that mindfulness usually fosters better social relationships. Since we spend so much time at work, getting on better with our colleagues will make the whole experience richer.

Above: Mindfulness not only improves work performance, but helps you enjoy your job more, too

APPEALING TO MEN

Given its proven benefits, it's important that mindfulness training is made more appealing to men. One way is to look at examples of mindfulness in practice. For example, a sprinter, standing at the start of the Olympic 100 metres, staring down the track and cocooned in concentration, is practising a form of mindfulness. The concentration, the focus on the moment, the relaxation, all help to bring an athlete to absolute peak performance. Understanding that mindfulness takes many forms and is practised by many of our role models makes it more accessible and appealing.

On a social level, having mindfulness classes led by men also improves male participation. Having a respected colleague or boss champion the practice of mindfulness will encourage other men to give it a try. Could it be you?

However, it must be pointed out that, like all psychological techniques, mindfulness is not a panacea for everybody. Making mindfulness training voluntary rather than mandatory also improves its continued implementation among male workers.

Mindfulness and emotional intelligence

How mindfulness can provide the 'x' factor for success

Multiple studies have shown that emotional intelligence – the ability to understand one's own emotions accurately and to respond appropriately to the emotions of other people – is one of the key factors in success in the workplace. This ability is often absolutely key both to making the best of one's own ability and to leading a team or organisation. As mindfulness produces greater appreciation of one's emotional states, it also facilitates greater understanding of the pressures and aims felt by other people in your organisation.

Mindfulness for Men

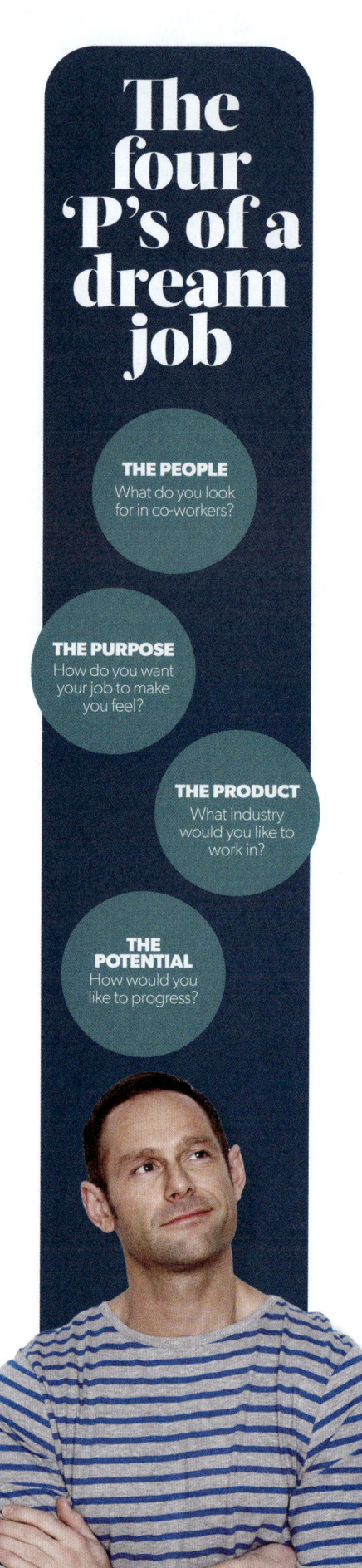

The four 'P's of a dream job

THE PEOPLE
What do you look for in co-workers?

THE PURPOSE
How do you want your job to make you feel?

THE PRODUCT
What industry would you like to work in?

THE POTENTIAL
How would you like to progress?

APPLYING MINDFULNESS TO YOUR CAREER

Within the context of the working day, the regular practice of mindfulness produces undeniable results for many men. But can we apply it towards a more holistic approach towards life and work? Many practitioners believe that we can. Mindfulness can first of all be employed to examine the day-to-day experience of one's work life. By focusing rigorously on the experience of the moment, it becomes much easier to sort out the stresses and strains that are intrinsic to the job and those that we bring to our career by our responses to people and situations. Doing so allows us to gather a much better impression of whether the job we are doing actually matches the ideals and aims one has in mind for the future.

Indeed, deciding one's overall career goal is a vital element of any successful career. Applying mindfulness techniques

SINGLE-TASK NOT MULTI-TASK

Multi-tasking is incompatible with a mindful outlook, as well as being inherently inefficient. Focus on one thing at a time.

to the examination of what we really want from a job enables us to focus on what really matters to us, rather than what our peers or wider society might expect of us.

To understand how to do this practically, suppose the boss calls you into their office and offers you a promotion to the new office in New York.

Faced with a momentous decision such as this, focusing on the present moment of reaction will provide an invaluable guide to its suitability. Not forcing emotions – faced with such an opportunity, it's easy to feel obligated to express delight and surprise – but rather viewing what your body and mind tell you in the moment will demonstrate your unfiltered reaction, while also enabling you to investigate whether parts of the reaction lie in perceptions of fear or inadequacy. But mindfulness is not only internal: it's your response to the person right in front of you. By focusing on the instant, you will be able to tell much about the way in which the job is being offered to you, whether gracefully and eagerly or because another candidate has already turned it down.

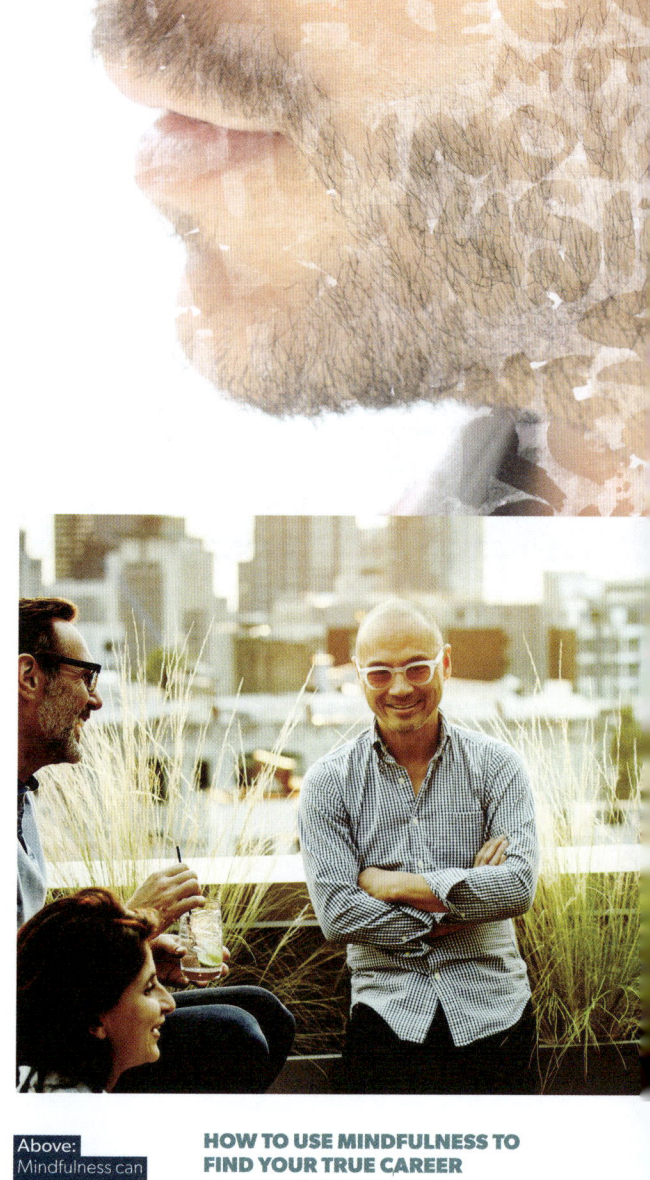

Above: Mindfulness can help you to get along better with the people with whom you work

HOW TO USE MINDFULNESS TO FIND YOUR TRUE CAREER

It's easy to drift into a career without thinking about whether it represents our true purpose in life. Society and peer pressure can take us in directions that we had no real intention of going in. One way of taking stock, when embarked upon a career path, is to write down what your career currently entails, what you'd really like to be doing (the two can be the same, of course), and any difficulties you

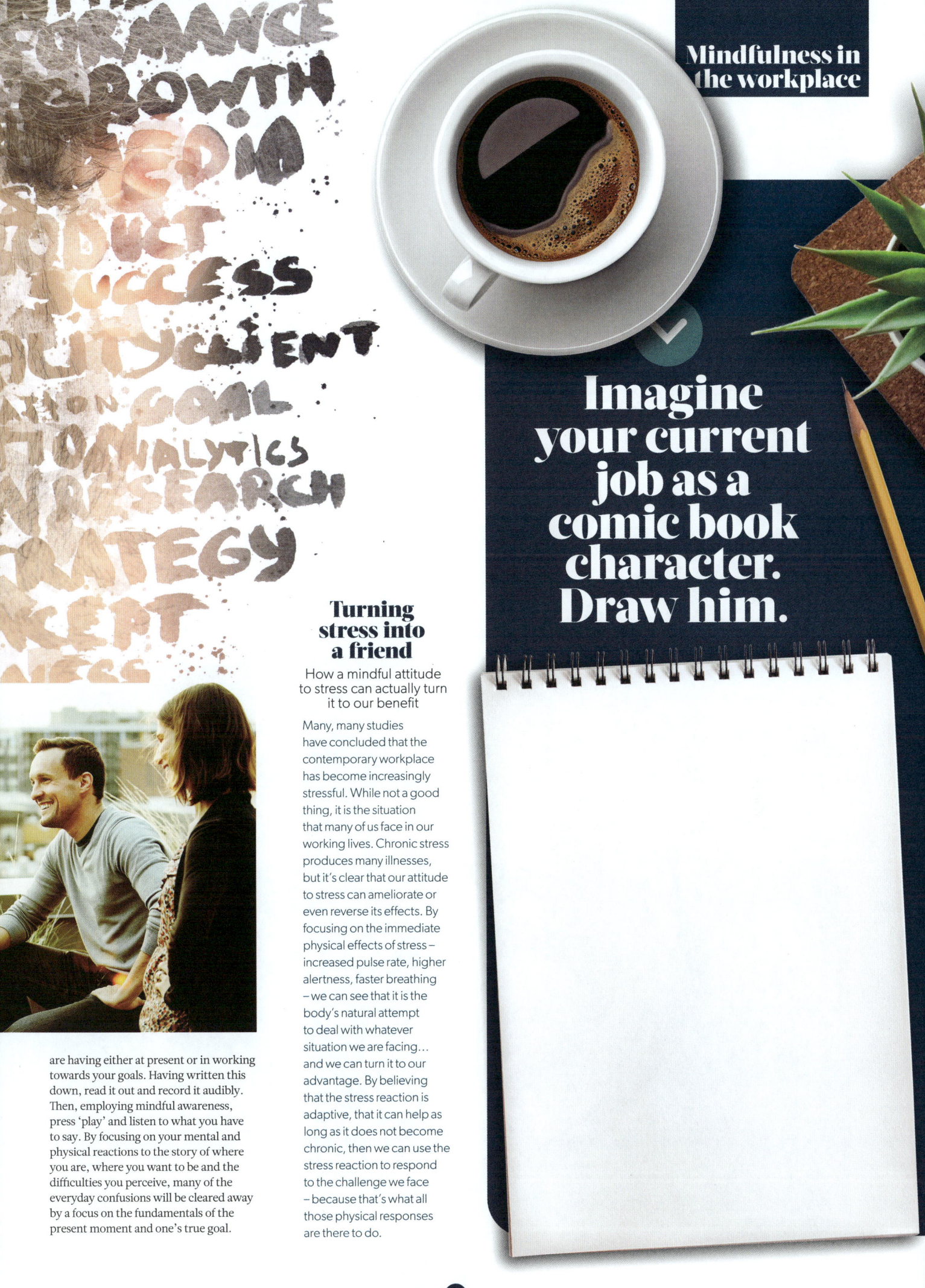

Mindfulness in the workplace

Imagine your current job as a comic book character. Draw him.

Turning stress into a friend

How a mindful attitude to stress can actually turn it to our benefit

Many, many studies have concluded that the contemporary workplace has become increasingly stressful. While not a good thing, it is the situation that many of us face in our working lives. Chronic stress produces many illnesses, but it's clear that our attitude to stress can ameliorate or even reverse its effects. By focusing on the immediate physical effects of stress – increased pulse rate, higher alertness, faster breathing – we can see that it is the body's natural attempt to deal with whatever situation we are facing… and we can turn it to our advantage. By believing that the stress reaction is adaptive, that it can help as long as it does not become chronic, then we can use the stress reaction to respond to the challenge we face – because that's what all those physical responses are there to do.

are having either at present or in working towards your goals. Having written this down, read it out and record it audibly. Then, employing mindful awareness, press 'play' and listen to what you have to say. By focusing on your mental and physical reactions to the story of where you are, where you want to be and the difficulties you perceive, many of the everyday confusions will be cleared away by a focus on the fundamentals of the present moment and one's true goal.

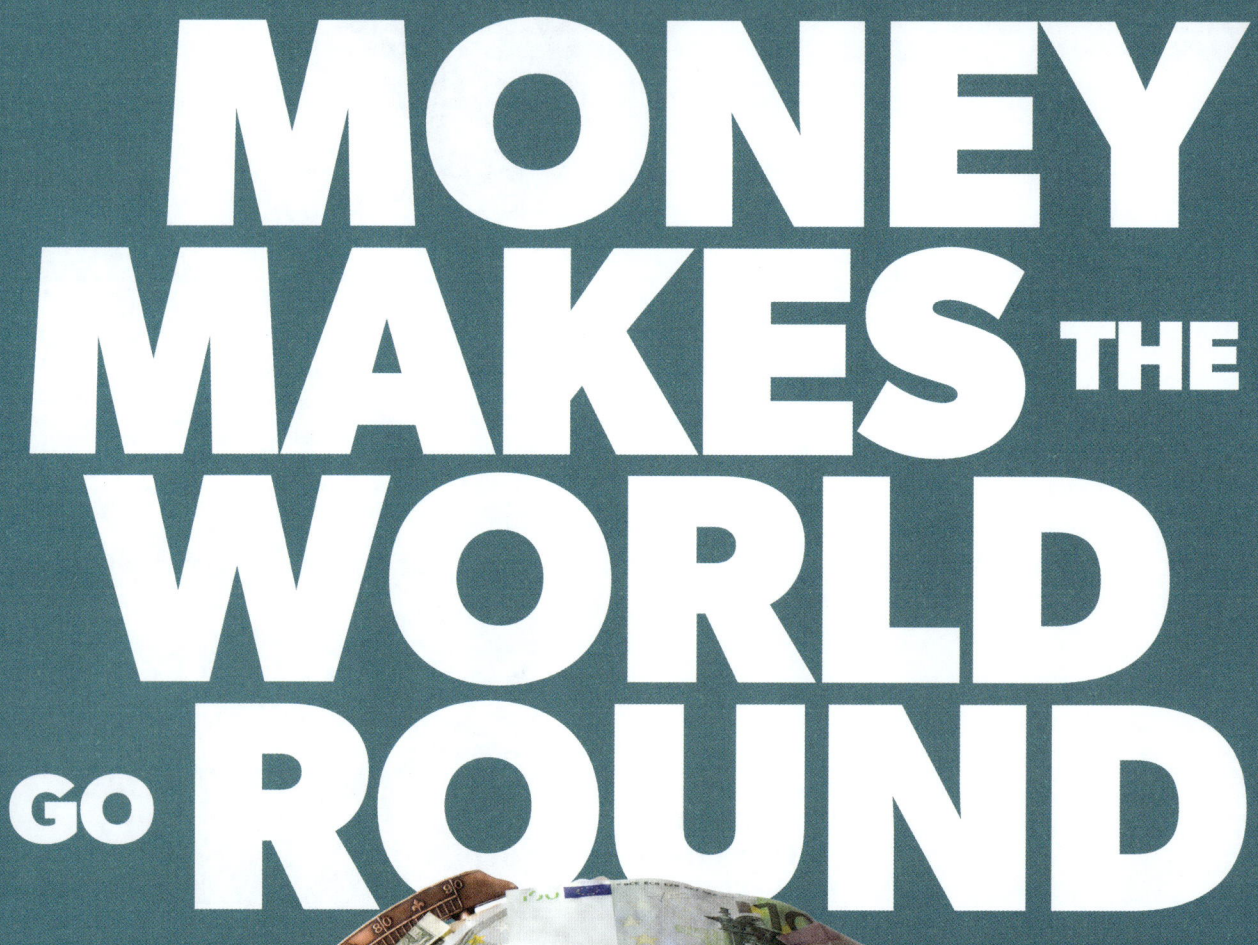

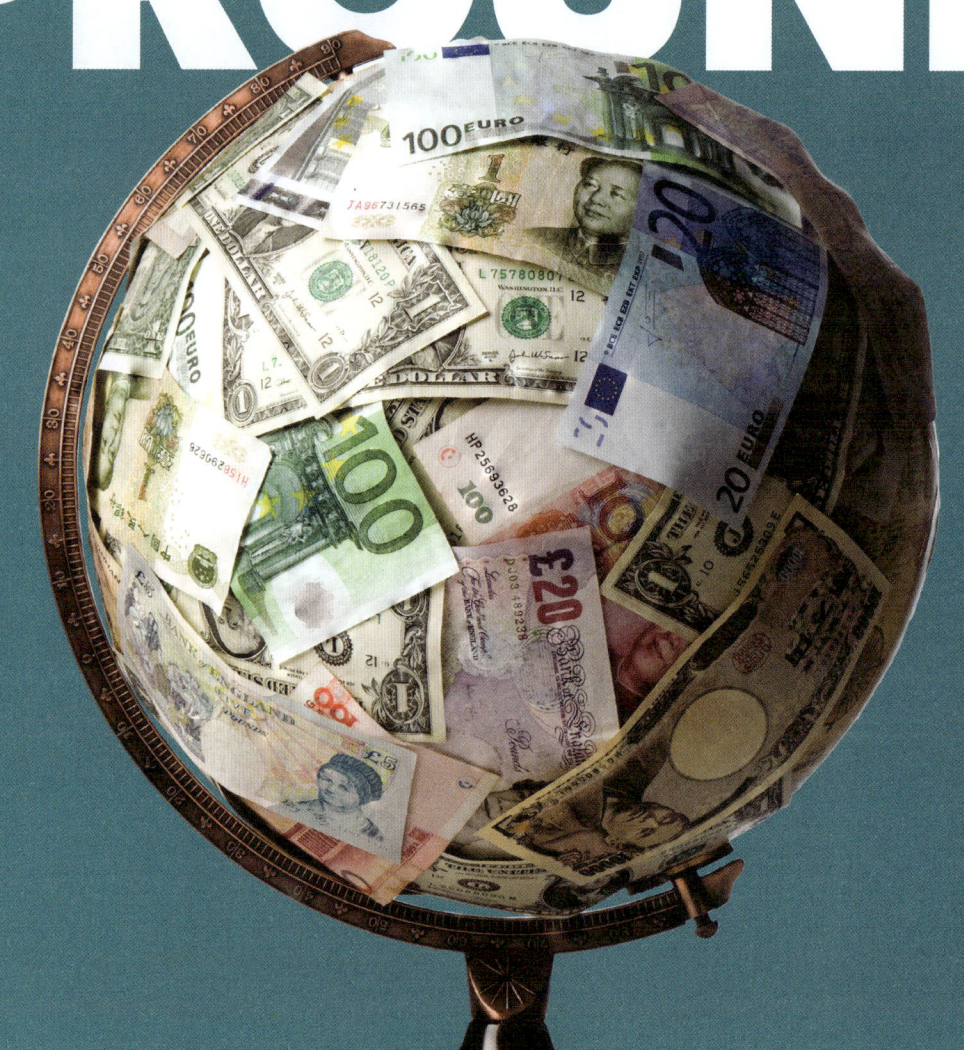

Mindfulness for Men

MONEY MAKES THE WORLD GO ROUND

Both the root of all evil and the grease that turns the wheels of the world, our relationship with money can be complicated, but it doesn't need to be…

> **Write down in the balloons what you would do with a million pounds should you win the lottery.**

Money can make us feel all kinds of emotions. Most of us have dreamed about what we'd spend it on if we were given a large sum unexpectedly, perhaps through a win or maybe as inheritance. However, the reality of being in this situation is likely to also cause a degree of stress or anxiety, sometimes even fear, particularly if we're not used to having a lot of money. Perhaps more relatable is the stress we feel when we struggle to make ends meet or can't afford little luxuries or treats. It can feel like a vicious cycle as sometimes we end up spending money we don't have in an attempt to seek emotional comfort. It could be a one-off big spend, such as a holiday or something for the home like a new TV. Or it could be smaller financial spends that occur more frequently, like nights out or ordering takeaways. These small purchases all add up.

Money does not equal happiness, but it can often break down barriers to enable us to do things that *do* make us happy. According to a survey by the Mental Health Foundation, 22% of people feeling stressed cited debt as a causing factor. Despite it being a problem, we don't talk as openly about our personal financial worries as we do with other aspects of our lives.

HOW WE LOOK AT MONEY
As much as we would like to avoid looking at our finances, and rather bury our heads in the sand, taking the time to see your money and analyse what is going on is key to having a healthy relationship with it. Take a moment to think about how you feel about money when you have it and if this has changed over time. What are your beliefs around money? How did or do your parents behave with their money? Do certain words such as 'budget' feel uncomfortable? What are your financial fears? When you spend money, how do you feel?

The first step to having a healthy relationship with your finances is to look at all of your income and outgoings, and we mean everything. Create a spreadsheet or find a budgeting app that works for you, and note down your salary, savings, credit cards, loans and so on. As you look at these, be mindful of how you're feeling. Does anything surprise you? Does anything leave that horrible feeling in your gut?

Remember that most of us worry about money from time to time. You are not alone. Some of us are even guilty of associating our income or financial position with our worth, and when we are having financial issues it can cause us to feel shame or guilt. But earning less than your partner or not having as much disposable income as your friends is not a reflection on you as a person or how successful you are, and doesn't dictate what people think of you. These feelings often rear their heads when we're invited somewhere and can't afford to go. There is no shame in admitting to friends that money is a bit tight or that you have other financial priorities. We've all been there, and it's possible that someone else in the group is grateful you've raised the issue, as they feel exactly the same.

MINDFUL SPENDING
With a lot of our daily monetary transactions taking place digitally, it can be difficult to get a grasp of what we are actually spending. If we handed over physical money for all of our subscriptions and purchases, would we

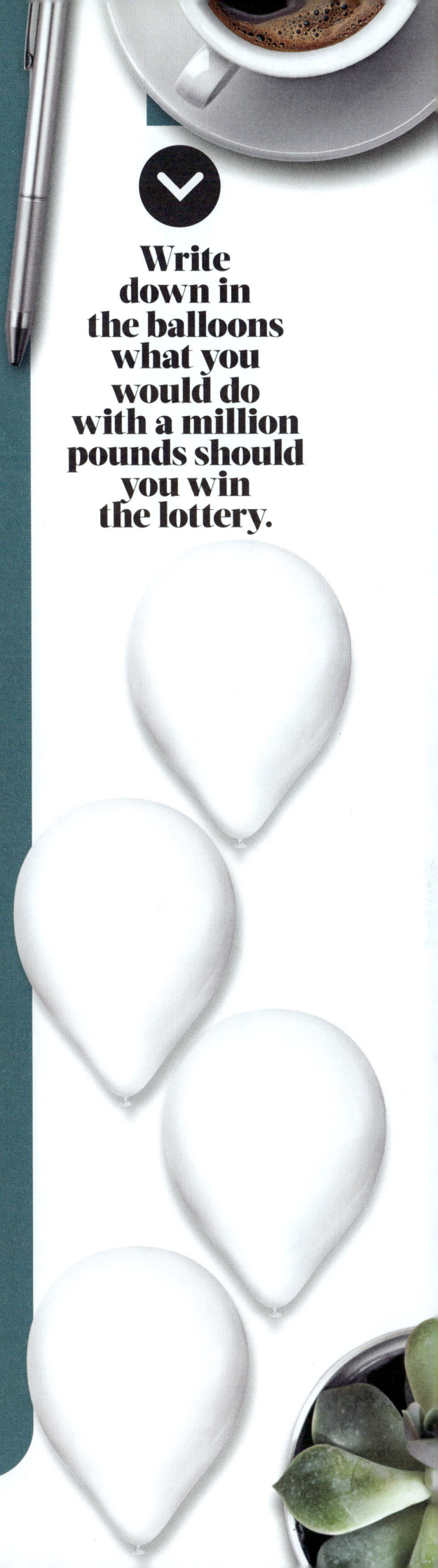

> **DON'T BE AN OSTRICH**
> The ostrich position – head down, stuck in the sand – is absolutely the worst way to deal with money, but shame or guilt means that many people adopt this position. Be mindful and stand up straight!

43

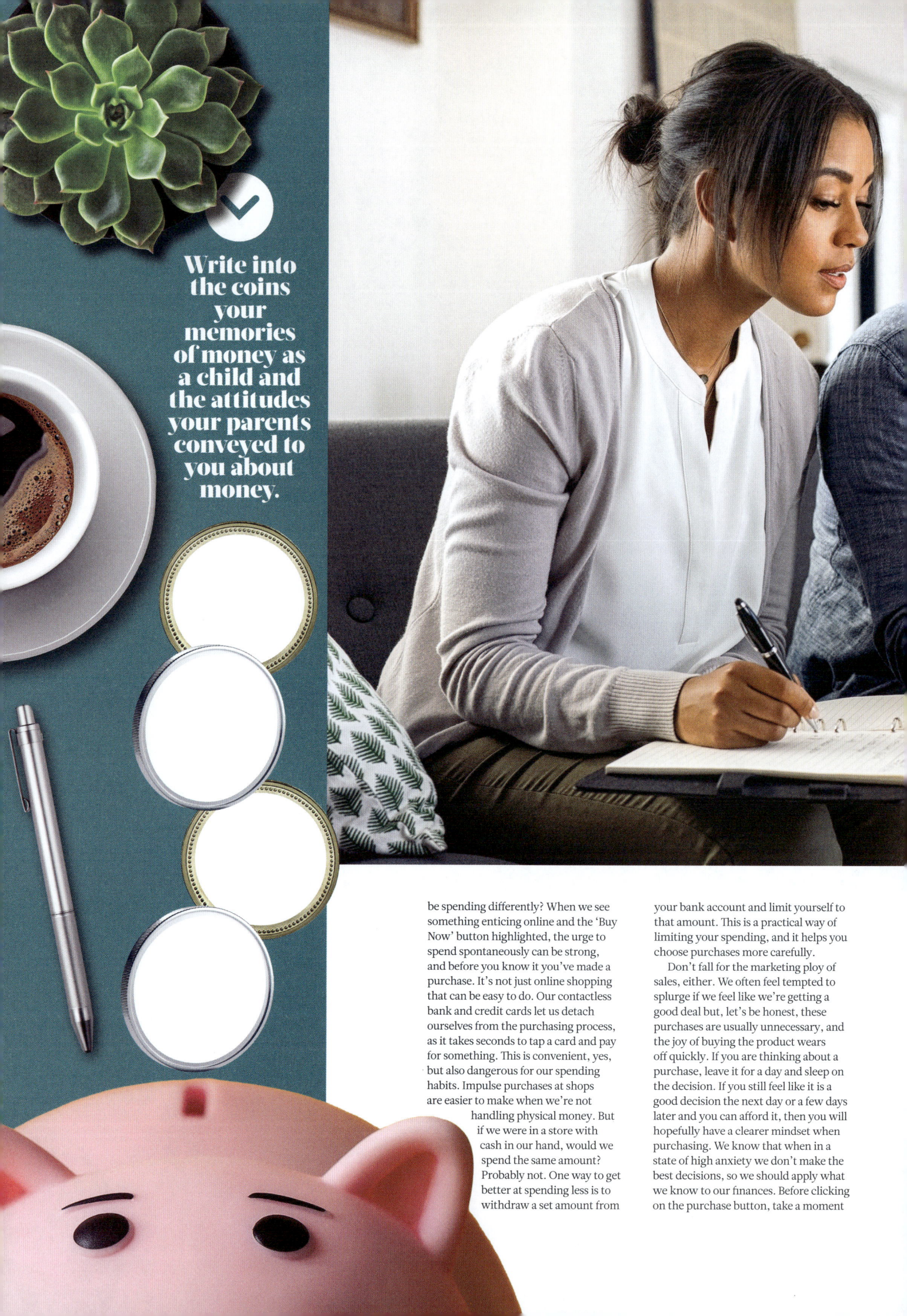

> Write into the coins your memories of money as a child and the attitudes your parents conveyed to you about money.

be spending differently? When we see something enticing online and the 'Buy Now' button highlighted, the urge to spend spontaneously can be strong, and before you know it you've made a purchase. It's not just online shopping that can be easy to do. Our contactless bank and credit cards let us detach ourselves from the purchasing process, as it takes seconds to tap a card and pay for something. This is convenient, yes, but also dangerous for our spending habits. Impulse purchases at shops are easier to make when we're not handling physical money. But if we were in a store with cash in our hand, would we spend the same amount? Probably not. One way to get better at spending less is to withdraw a set amount from your bank account and limit yourself to that amount. This is a practical way of limiting your spending, and it helps you choose purchases more carefully.

Don't fall for the marketing ploy of sales, either. We often feel tempted to splurge if we feel like we're getting a good deal but, let's be honest, these purchases are usually unnecessary, and the joy of buying the product wears off quickly. If you are thinking about a purchase, leave it for a day and sleep on the decision. If you still feel like it is a good decision the next day or a few days later and you can afford it, then you will hopefully have a clearer mindset when purchasing. We know that when in a state of high anxiety we don't make the best decisions, so we should apply what we know to our finances. Before clicking on the purchase button, take a moment

Money makes the world go round

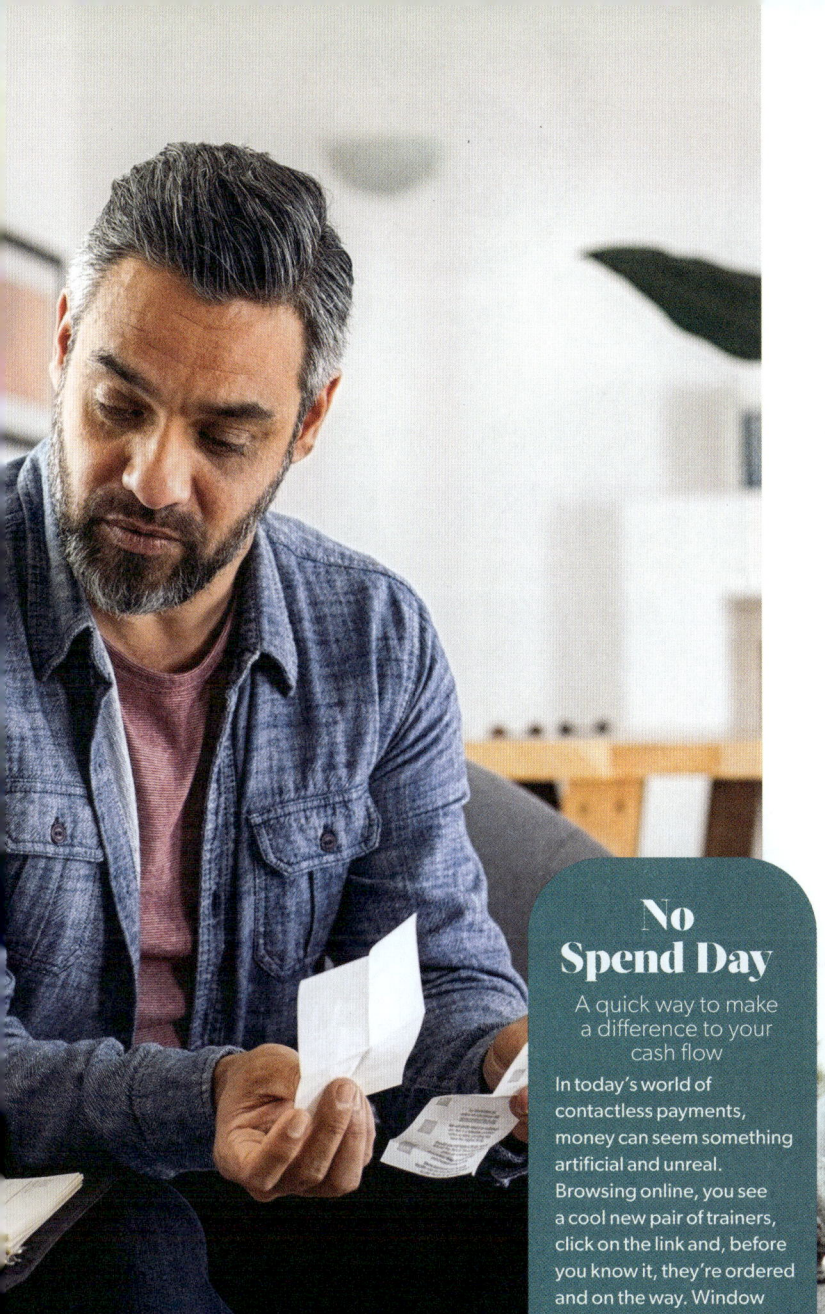

Left: Keep an eye on your outgoings every day, not just when you get bank notifications

pick it up later when you need it or are in a better financial position.

HOW TO MAKE A KAKEIBO
Many households in Japan use a system called 'kakeibo', which was developed in the early 1900s. The word translates to 'household finance book', and was originally meant to enable homemakers to see their family's spending habits and help control finances. To make your own kakeibo, you must answer four simple questions: How much money do you have coming in? How much do you want to save? How much do you spend? How can this be improved?

The first step is to write down how much money you have coming in at the start of each month, and subtract your fixed expenses such as rent and bills. Now set a goal of how much money you

to breathe and connect with yourself. Taking the time to do this can help avoid self-destructive behaviour, such as spending money you don't have.

Changing your habits around viewing your bank balance can remove some of your financial stress. If you only check your bank account when you need to pay an urgent bill and you do it grudgingly, then you will likely keep a negative attitude towards your money. With bank apps available on smartphones, you can keep on top of your balance easily. Regular checks can also help to avoid problems from becoming neglected and growing. Regularly check direct debits and outgoings to see if they're all necessary. Do you need multiple subscriptions to streaming services? If you know you won't be using one for some time, cancel the subscription and

No Spend Day
A quick way to make a difference to your cash flow

In today's world of contactless payments, money can seem something artificial and unreal. Browsing online, you see a cool new pair of trainers, click on the link and, before you know it, they're ordered and on the way. Window shopping, you see that the new *Call of Duty* game is out. A touch on the card reader and the game is yours. Modern culture is geared towards making it swift and easy to buy things. The pain comes later. To start making an immediate, tangible difference to your cash flow, decide upon a No Spend Day. This is a day when you will spend money only on the essentials: the train fare to work, maybe lunch at work (although you could take in a packed lunch), the fare home. No impulse purchase in the supermarket. No expensive treat as a self-reward for doing an hour in the gym. A mindful No Spend Day is an excellent way of identifying triggers to unconscious spending, as well as a way of immediately reducing your outgoings.

Bad habits

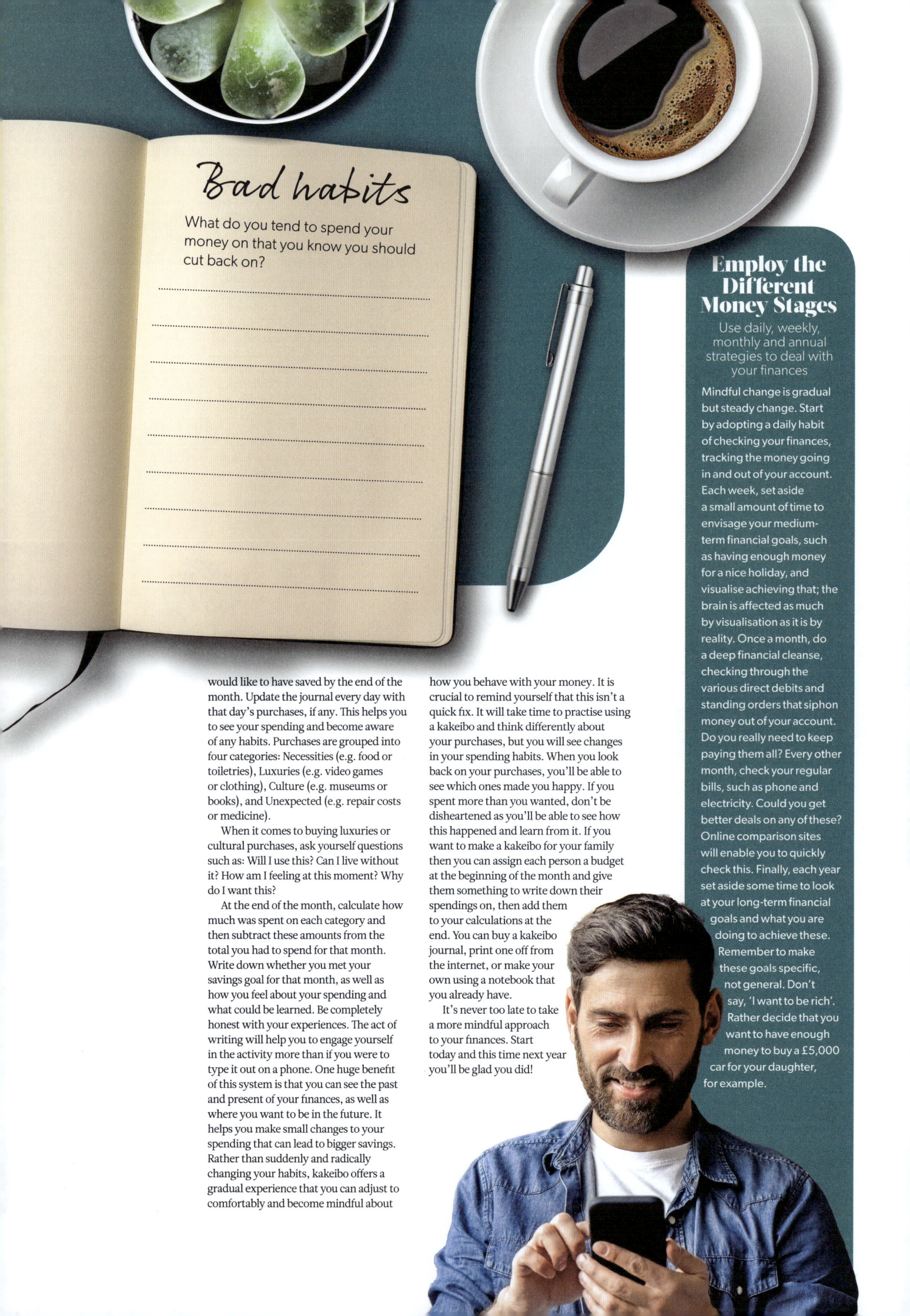

What do you tend to spend your money on that you know you should cut back on?

....
....
....
....
....
....
....

would like to have saved by the end of the month. Update the journal every day with that day's purchases, if any. This helps you to see your spending and become aware of any habits. Purchases are grouped into four categories: Necessities (e.g. food or toiletries), Luxuries (e.g. video games or clothing), Culture (e.g. museums or books), and Unexpected (e.g. repair costs or medicine).

When it comes to buying luxuries or cultural purchases, ask yourself questions such as: Will I use this? Can I live without it? How am I feeling at this moment? Why do I want this?

At the end of the month, calculate how much was spent on each category and then subtract these amounts from the total you had to spend for that month. Write down whether you met your savings goal for that month, as well as how you feel about your spending and what could be learned. Be completely honest with your experiences. The act of writing will help you to engage yourself in the activity more than if you were to type it out on a phone. One huge benefit of this system is that you can see the past and present of your finances, as well as where you want to be in the future. It helps you make small changes to your spending that can lead to bigger savings. Rather than suddenly and radically changing your habits, kakeibo offers a gradual experience that you can adjust to comfortably and become mindful about how you behave with your money. It is crucial to remind yourself that this isn't a quick fix. It will take time to practise using a kakeibo and think differently about your purchases, but you will see changes in your spending habits. When you look back on your purchases, you'll be able to see which ones made you happy. If you spent more than you wanted, don't be disheartened as you'll be able to see how this happened and learn from it. If you want to make a kakeibo for your family then you can assign each person a budget at the beginning of the month and give them something to write down their spendings on, then add them to your calculations at the end. You can buy a kakeibo journal, print one off from the internet, or make your own using a notebook that you already have.

It's never too late to take a more mindful approach to your finances. Start today and this time next year you'll be glad you did!

Employ the Different Money Stages

Use daily, weekly, monthly and annual strategies to deal with your finances

Mindful change is gradual but steady change. Start by adopting a daily habit of checking your finances, tracking the money going in and out of your account. Each week, set aside a small amount of time to envisage your medium-term financial goals, such as having enough money for a nice holiday, and visualise achieving that; the brain is affected as much by visualisation as it is by reality. Once a month, do a deep financial cleanse, checking through the various direct debits and standing orders that siphon money out of your account. Do you really need to keep paying them all? Every other month, check your regular bills, such as phone and electricity. Could you get better deals on any of these? Online comparison sites will enable you to quickly check this. Finally, each year set aside some time to look at your long-term financial goals and what you are doing to achieve these. Remember to make these goals specific, not general. Don't say, 'I want to be rich'. Rather decide that you want to have enough money to buy a £5,000 car for your daughter, for example.

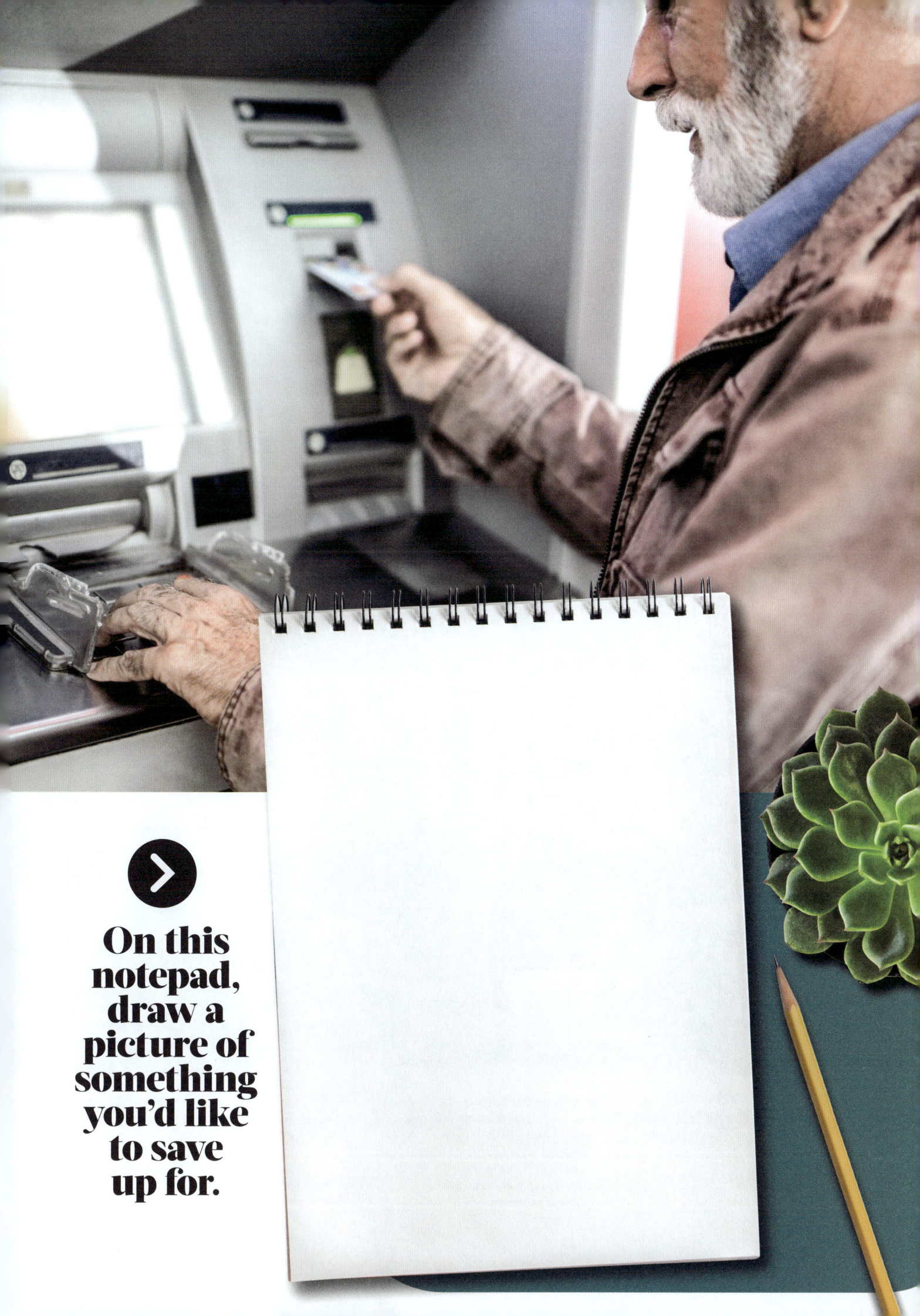

> **On this notepad, draw a picture of something you'd like to save up for.**

Mindfulness for Men

HOBBIES AND INTERESTS

Engaging mindfully in hobbies that you enjoy can reap huge benefits for your mental health and wellbeing

5 ways to make space for your hobbies
Do you feel like you're just too busy to take up a hobby? Here are some top tips to help prioritise your interests

1 DIARISE YOUR HOBBIES
Make an appointment with your hobby, whether that's a fixed training session or a specific time to do your hobby. Put it in your calendar to give it the same importance as other areas of your life.

2 INVOLVE OTHERS
Can you share your hobby with other people in your life? If you like walking, for example, can you make it a family activity that you can all enjoy together?

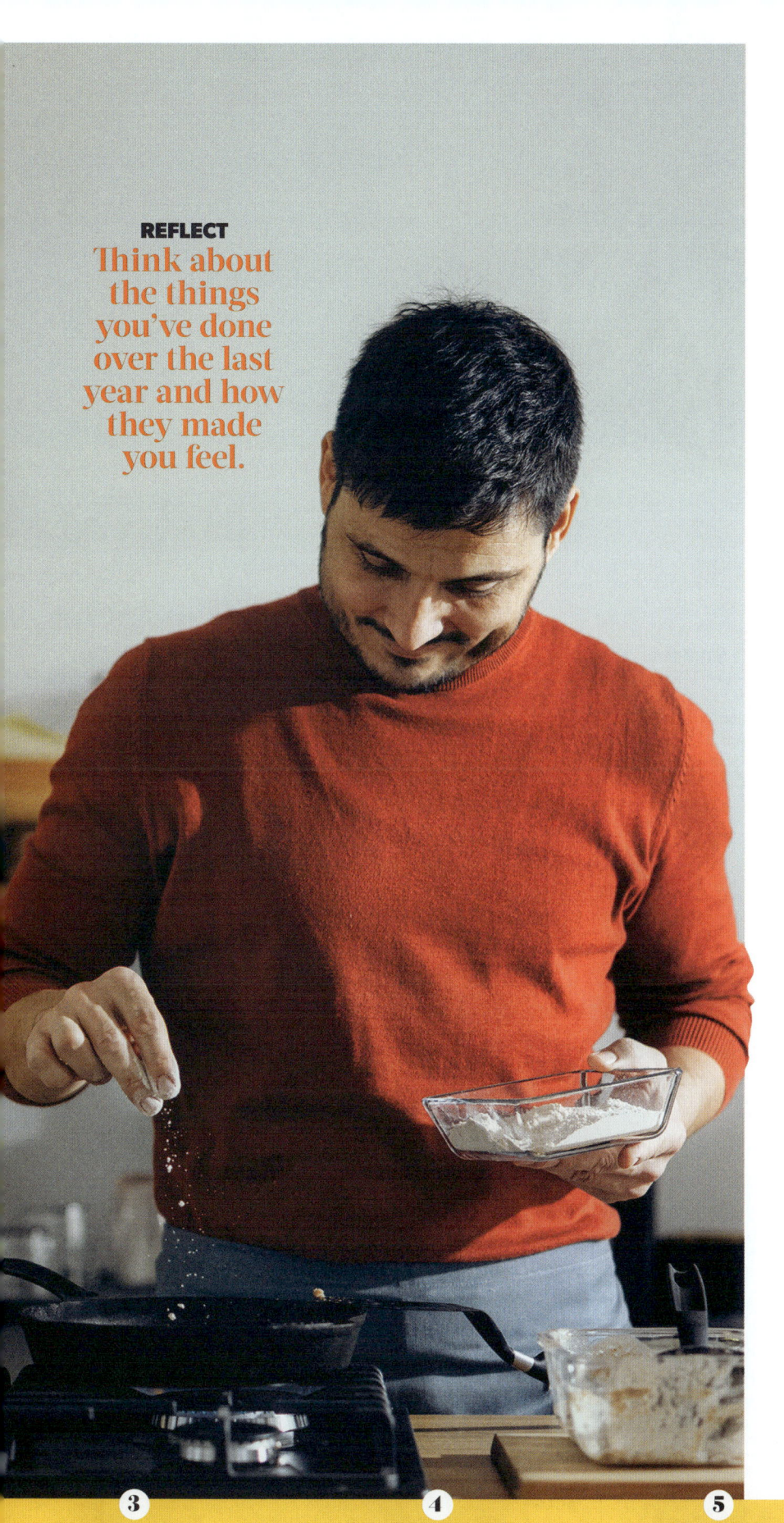

Hobbies and interests

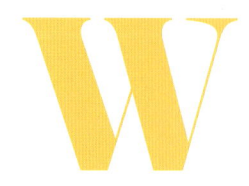

REFLECT
Think about the things you've done over the last year and how they made you feel.

When day-to-day life is busy, with work, family commitments or life admin, it's so easy to spend any downtime watching television or trying to catch up on missed chores. Hobbies can be seen as an indulgence, something to do when and if you have the time. However, having a hobby or interest is good for your mental health and wellbeing, and also gives you the perfect opportunity to practise mindfulness regularly. So it's worthwhile making space in your life for a hobby or two, even if only for a short amount of time each week.

Hobbies are very personal. A hobby is 'an activity done regularly in leisure time for pleasure'. There are two key components to this definition to be aware of. First, a hobby should be something that brings you joy – there's no point taking part in something you don't enjoy and doesn't give you pleasure. Sometimes we do activities because we feel we should, or because we've done them for a long time, or because they make someone else happy. But, be honest with yourself, do the activities you choose to do in your leisure time make you truly happy?

The second element is that your hobby should be done regularly – this means actively making time to participate in your chosen hobby routinely, and not just now and then. It's something that should form part of your weekly routine, rather than an afterthought if you want to really feel the benefits.

CHOOSING A HOBBY
You may already have a hobby that you enjoy – whether that's taking part in a sport, cooking, reading or developing a skill, for example. That's great! Finding the right hobby to suit you can be the first hurdle to overcome. If you have a hobby you love, then think about whether you give it enough

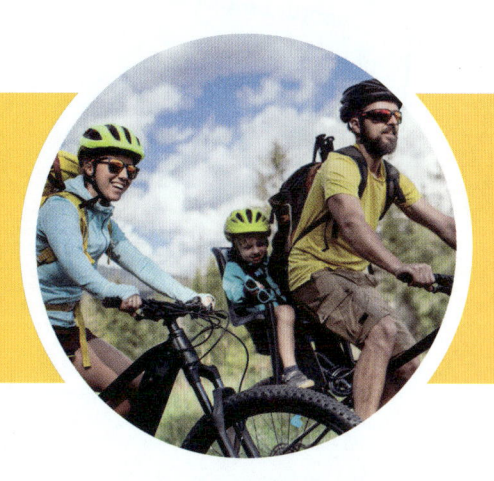

3
SET A GOAL
Having a specific goal or target can help you to stay motivated and make more time for your interests.

4
BE CREATIVE WITH YOUR TIME
How can you fit your hobby into your life in different ways? If you like cycling, can you commute to work by bike? If you enjoy drawing, can you carry a sketchbook in your bag to doodle in your lunchbreak?

5
JOIN A GROUP
Having other people to meet makes it easier to find time to do your hobby. Have a look in your local community for shared interest groups.

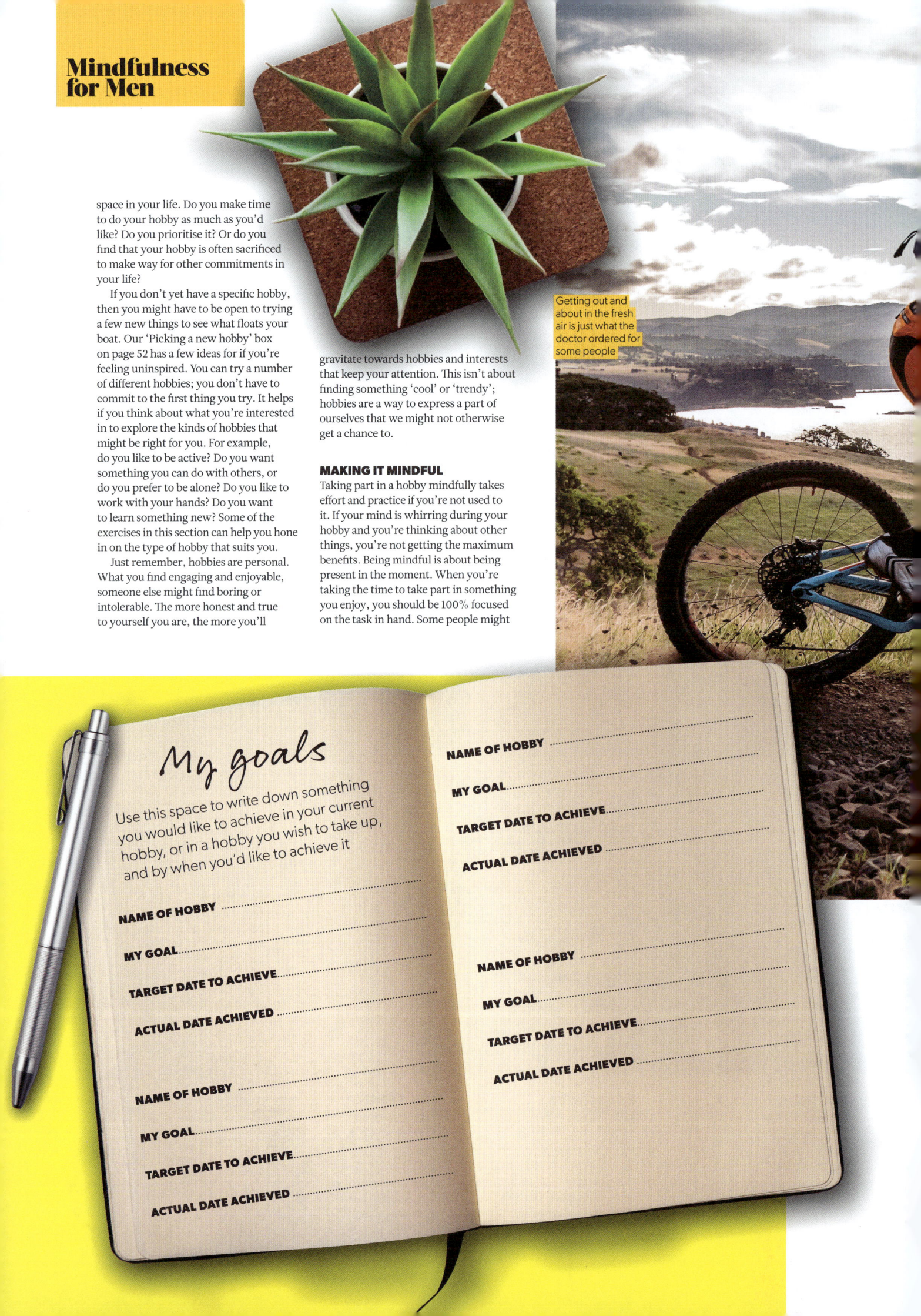

Mindfulness for Men

space in your life. Do you make time to do your hobby as much as you'd like? Do you prioritise it? Or do you find that your hobby is often sacrificed to make way for other commitments in your life?

If you don't yet have a specific hobby, then you might have to be open to trying a few new things to see what floats your boat. Our 'Picking a new hobby' box on page 52 has a few ideas for if you're feeling uninspired. You can try a number of different hobbies; you don't have to commit to the first thing you try. It helps if you think about what you're interested in to explore the kinds of hobbies that might be right for you. For example, do you like to be active? Do you want something you can do with others, or do you prefer to be alone? Do you like to work with your hands? Do you want to learn something new? Some of the exercises in this section can help you hone in on the type of hobby that suits you.

Just remember, hobbies are personal. What you find engaging and enjoyable, someone else might find boring or intolerable. The more honest and true to yourself you are, the more you'll gravitate towards hobbies and interests that keep your attention. This isn't about finding something 'cool' or 'trendy'; hobbies are a way to express a part of ourselves that we might not otherwise get a chance to.

MAKING IT MINDFUL

Taking part in a hobby mindfully takes effort and practice if you're not used to it. If your mind is whirring during your hobby and you're thinking about other things, you're not getting the maximum benefits. Being mindful is about being present in the moment. When you're taking the time to take part in something you enjoy, you should be 100% focused on the task in hand. Some people might

Getting out and about in the fresh air is just what the doctor ordered for some people

My goals

Use this space to write down something you would like to achieve in your current hobby, or in a hobby you wish to take up, and by when you'd like to achieve it

NAME OF HOBBY ....

MY GOAL ....

TARGET DATE TO ACHIEVE ....

ACTUAL DATE ACHIEVED ....

NAME OF HOBBY ....

MY GOAL ....

TARGET DATE TO ACHIEVE ....

ACTUAL DATE ACHIEVED ....

NAME OF HOBBY ....

MY GOAL ....

TARGET DATE TO ACHIEVE ....

ACTUAL DATE ACHIEVED ....

NAME OF HOBBY ....

MY GOAL ....

TARGET DATE TO ACHIEVE ....

ACTUAL DATE ACHIEVED ....

Reflection

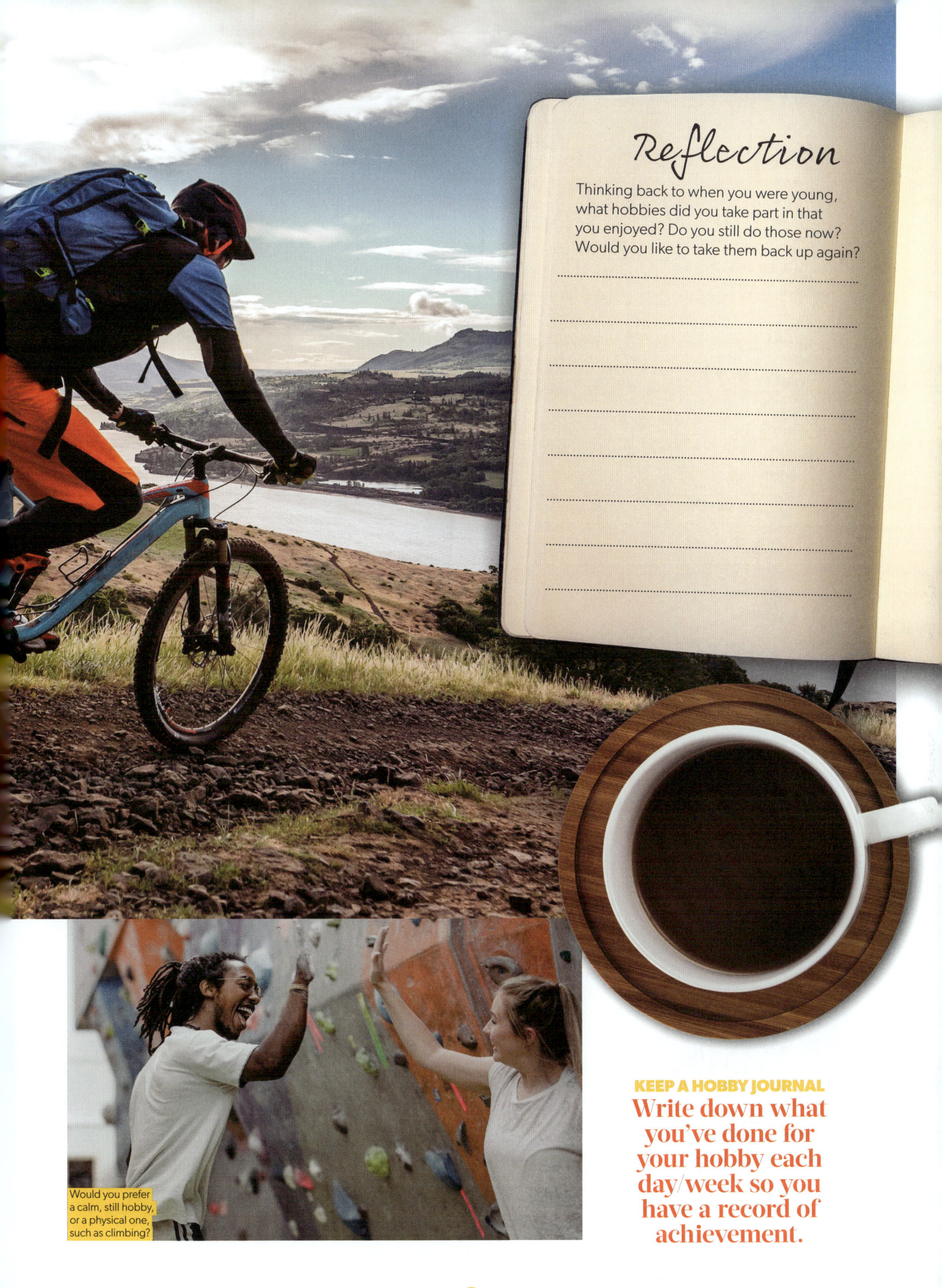

Thinking back to when you were young, what hobbies did you take part in that you enjoyed? Do you still do those now? Would you like to take them back up again?

....
....
....
....
....
....
....
....

Would you prefer a calm, still hobby, or a physical one, such as climbing?

KEEP A HOBBY JOURNAL
Write down what you've done for your hobby each day/week so you have a record of achievement.

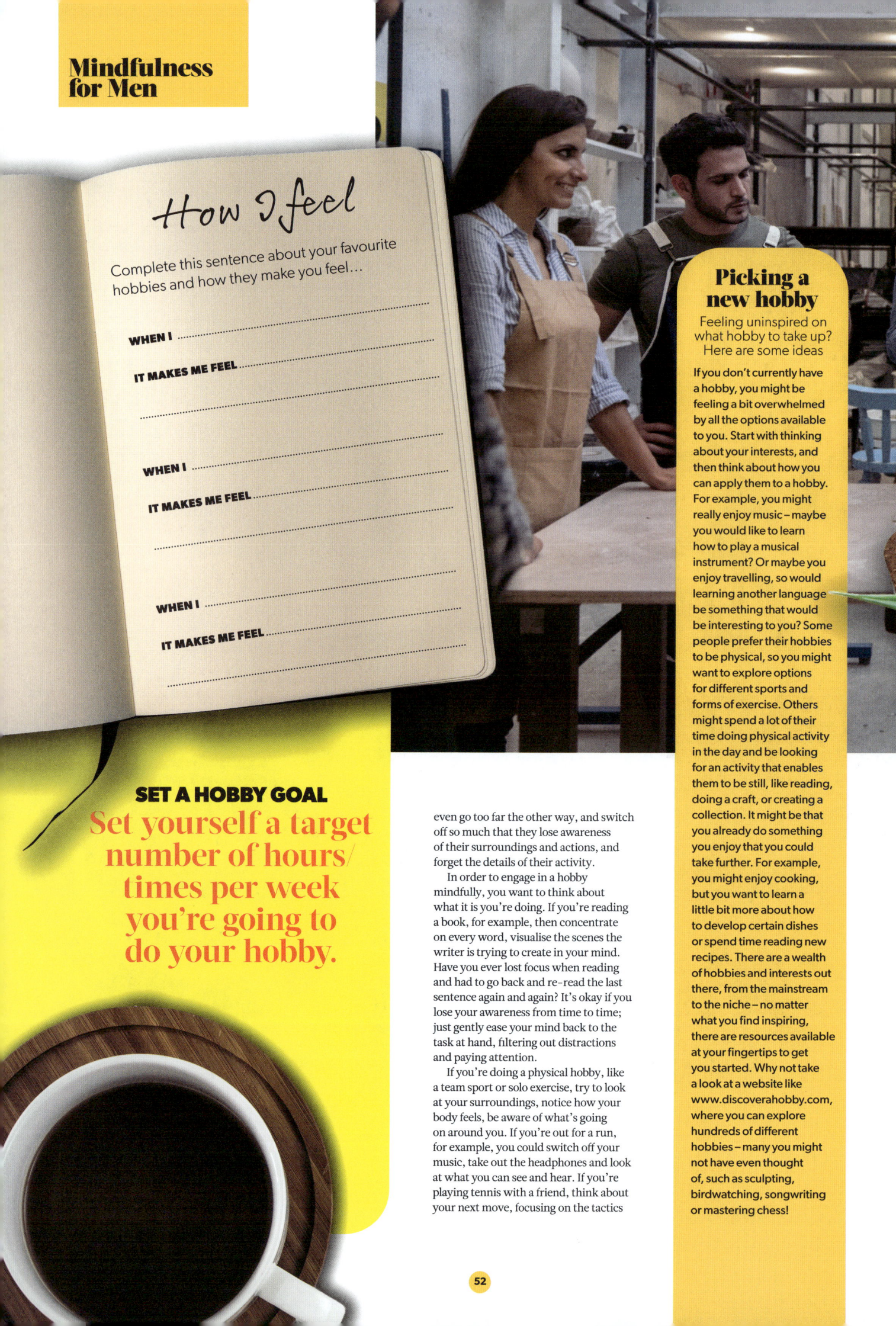

Mindfulness for Men

How I feel

Complete this sentence about your favourite hobbies and how they make you feel…

WHEN I ....

IT MAKES ME FEEL ....

....

WHEN I ....

IT MAKES ME FEEL ....

....

WHEN I ....

IT MAKES ME FEEL ....

....

SET A HOBBY GOAL

Set yourself a target number of hours/times per week you're going to do your hobby.

even go too far the other way, and switch off so much that they lose awareness of their surroundings and actions, and forget the details of their activity.

In order to engage in a hobby mindfully, you want to think about what it is you're doing. If you're reading a book, for example, then concentrate on every word, visualise the scenes the writer is trying to create in your mind. Have you ever lost focus when reading and had to go back and re-read the last sentence again and again? It's okay if you lose your awareness from time to time; just gently ease your mind back to the task at hand, filtering out distractions and paying attention.

If you're doing a physical hobby, like a team sport or solo exercise, try to look at your surroundings, notice how your body feels, be aware of what's going on around you. If you're out for a run, for example, you could switch off your music, take out the headphones and look at what you can see and hear. If you're playing tennis with a friend, think about your next move, focusing on the tactics

Picking a new hobby

Feeling uninspired on what hobby to take up? Here are some ideas

If you don't currently have a hobby, you might be feeling a bit overwhelmed by all the options available to you. Start with thinking about your interests, and then think about how you can apply them to a hobby. For example, you might really enjoy music – maybe you would like to learn how to play a musical instrument? Or maybe you enjoy travelling, so would learning another language be something that would be interesting to you? Some people prefer their hobbies to be physical, so you might want to explore options for different sports and forms of exercise. Others might spend a lot of their time doing physical activity in the day and be looking for an activity that enables them to be still, like reading, doing a craft, or creating a collection. It might be that you already do something you enjoy that you could take further. For example, you might enjoy cooking, but you want to learn a little bit more about how to develop certain dishes or spend time reading new recipes. There are a wealth of hobbies and interests out there, from the mainstream to the niche – no matter what you find inspiring, there are resources available at your fingertips to get you started. Why not take a look at a website like www.discoverahobby.com, where you can explore hundreds of different hobbies – many you might not have even thought of, such as sculpting, birdwatching, songwriting or mastering chess!

Hobbies and interests

My interests

Use this space to list down everything you're interested in, no matter how small or obscure, as this may inspire you to take up new hobbies in the future

- ....
- ....
- ....
- ....
- ....
- ....
- ....
- ....

and anticipating your opponent to help you stay in the moment.

THE BENEFITS OF HOBBIES
There are so many benefits of having a hobby, which are increased by engaging with the hobby in a mindful manner.

For a start, having a personal hobby can help you to feel more fulfilled in your life. Hobbies offer us a chance to progress in something, and improve, which triggers the body's reward response. We feel a sense of achievement, which in turn makes us feel good about ourselves. This can improve confidence and self-esteem, in both the hobby itself and in our wider life.

Hobbies can improve our wellbeing, and have been shown to help relieve the symptoms of stress, anxiety and depression. So much so, that in some areas, social prescribing is used to help those living with a mental health condition, where people are supported to attend things like gardening clubs or fitness groups.

Being mindfully focused on a hobby can also help to improve your concentration skills and memory. Rather than letting your mind wander, keeping in the moment helps you to give your brain a workout. This can then go on to benefit you in your personal and professional life, helping you feel sharper and more focused. Keeping the brain active may also help reduce the risk of developing dementia in later life by retaining healthy brain function.

Depending on your chosen hobby, it can also help you to be social and make new friends. If your hobby can be done in a group, it can help you to bond with likeminded souls over a shared interest. Even if your hobby is very much a solo endeavour, you may find chat groups online, for example, where you can discuss your interests and share tips. This social connection can also have great benefits for your mental health.

There is some science behind the reasons why hobbies are so beneficial. When we take part in an activity that we enjoy, our brain releases feel-good chemicals, such as dopamine, which make us feel pleasure and happiness. That feeling then helps act as motivation for us to do it again, to get another kick of dopamine. If we continue with our hobby regularly, we're feeding our brain with lots of happy hormones.

This can then have a big impact outside of our hobbies too. When we've given some time to our own pleasure and interests, we find it easier to engage with other areas of our lives. Having a hobby can help to improve our relationships with family, a partner or friends; it can help us to cope better with stress; it can help to find that perfect work-life balance; and it can help us feel generally happier and more content.

Taking time for a hobby doesn't come naturally for all of us. We might feel like we're being selfish to dedicate time to something we do purely for our own enjoyment, but not having something for ourselves can lead to feelings of resentment, unhappiness and loneliness. So remember that having a hobby you can mindfully partake in is a form of self-care, one that will help you to live a happier and more fulfilled life.

Above left: Joining a regular class is a great way to meet likeminded people, as well as learn a fun new skill

Mindfulness for Men

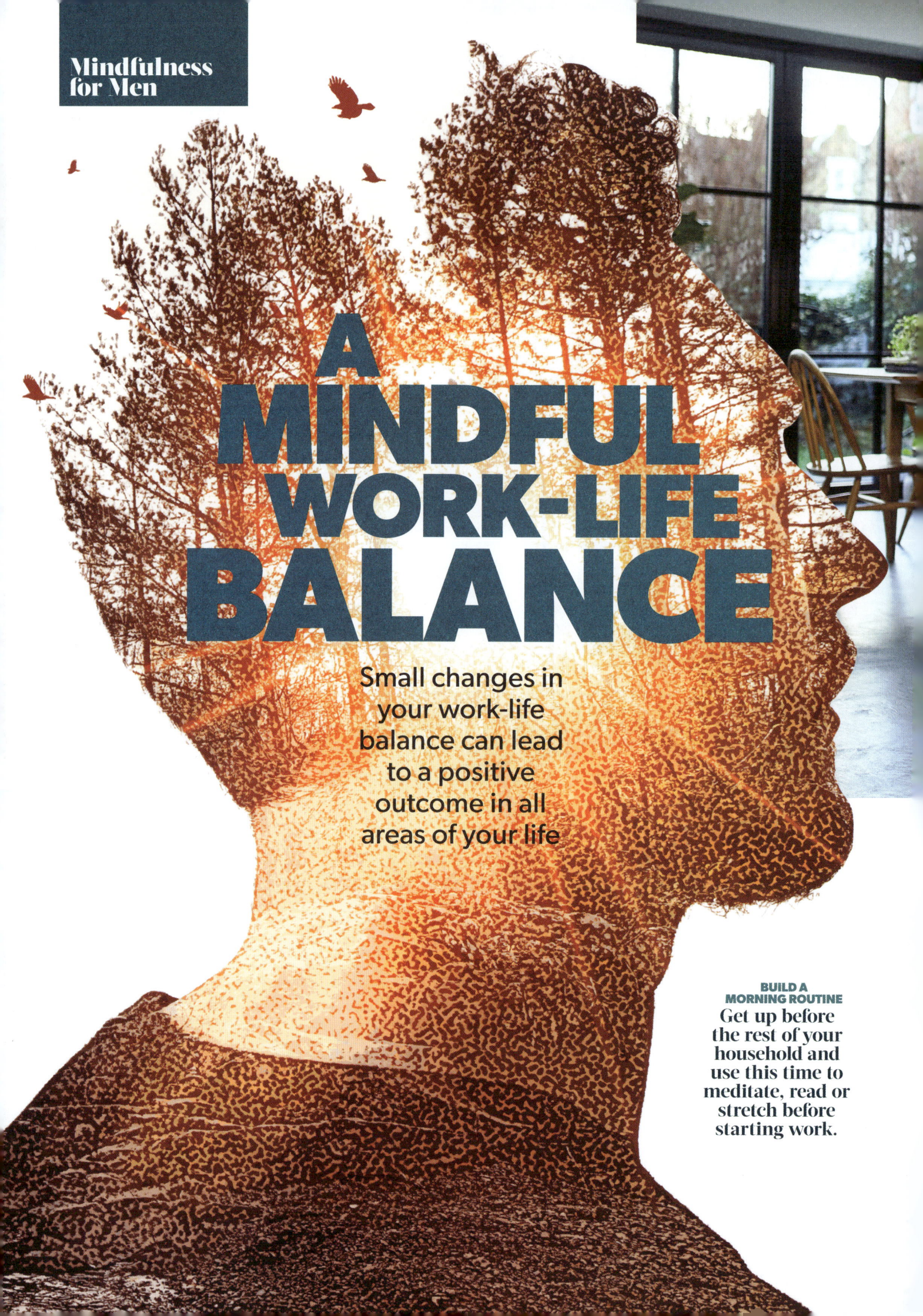

A MINDFUL WORK-LIFE BALANCE

Small changes in your work-life balance can lead to a positive outcome in all areas of your life

BUILD A MORNING ROUTINE
Get up before the rest of your household and use this time to meditate, read or stretch before starting work.

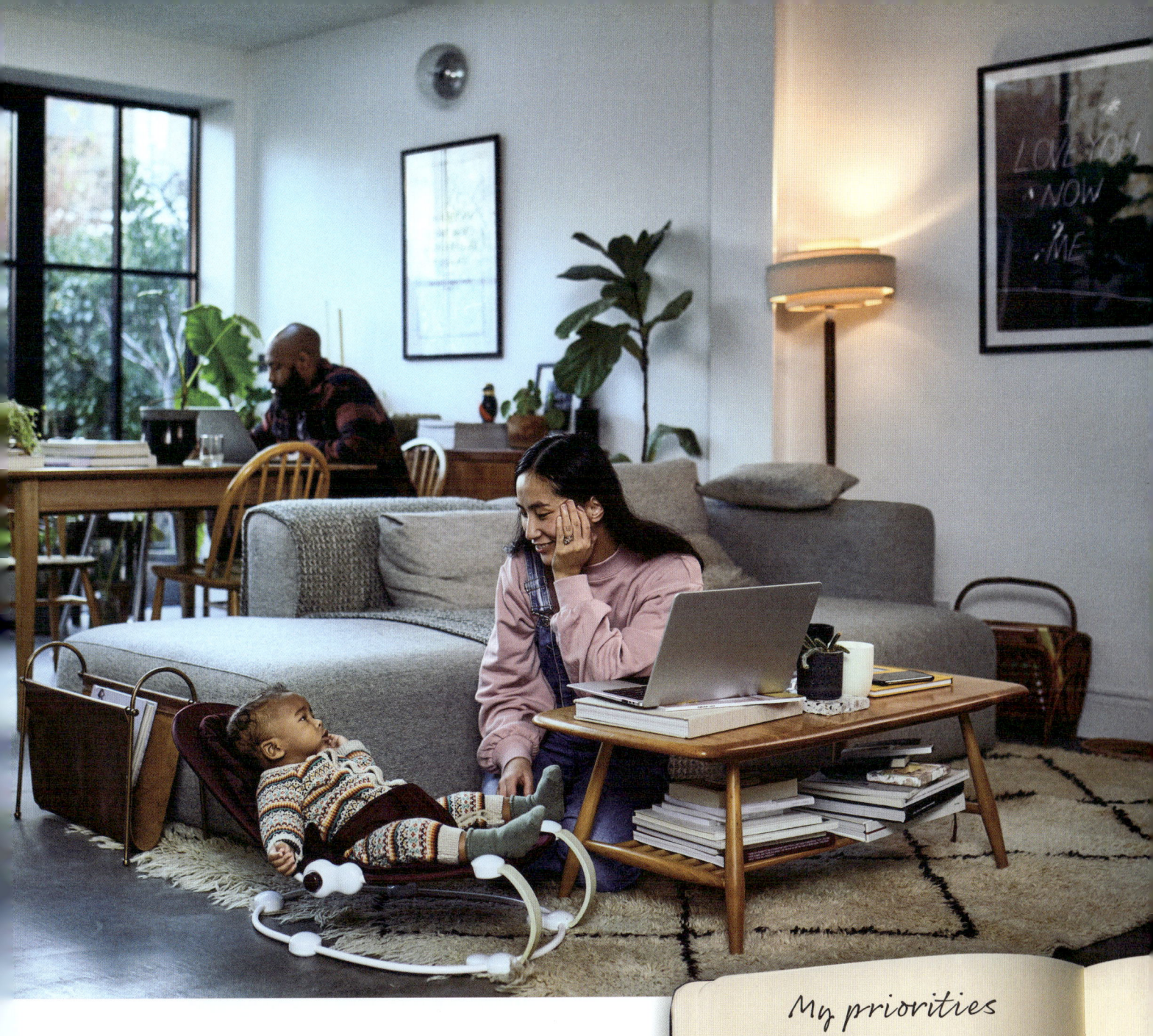

I f you're constantly feeling under pressure, stressed, short on time and overwhelmed, it could be because you have a work-life balance that isn't supporting your wellbeing. It's easy to let things build up and feel busy all the time, and yet not feel like there is any space in your life to do the things that you enjoy or spend time with the people you care about.

We're in a culture where busyness can often be seen as a desirable trait. We consider being busy at work as a sign of success; being socially busy makes us seem popular; and we might feel busy at home trying to keep on top of chores, responsibilities and life admin.

But being busy and on the go all the time can mean that we don't have time in our life for the things that we truly enjoy and that bring us joy. When the work-life balance is tipped towards work, you may be more prone to having low mental health; to having lower physical health if you're not making time to exercise; you might make poorer decisions around nutrition or alcohol intake; and your relationships could suffer if you're not spending enough time with family and friends.

Therefore, it pays to be mindful of your work-life balance – to be able to look at your current balance and see where you could make changes, and what would make you feel happier and more content. In this feature, we'll look at what a good work-life balance means and how to achieve the right balance for you.

My priorities

Use this space to write down your priorities in a typical day, whether that's spending time with friends/family, exercising, engaging in a hobby, getting more sleep and so on.

1 ....

2 ....

3 ....

4 ....

5 ....

6 ....

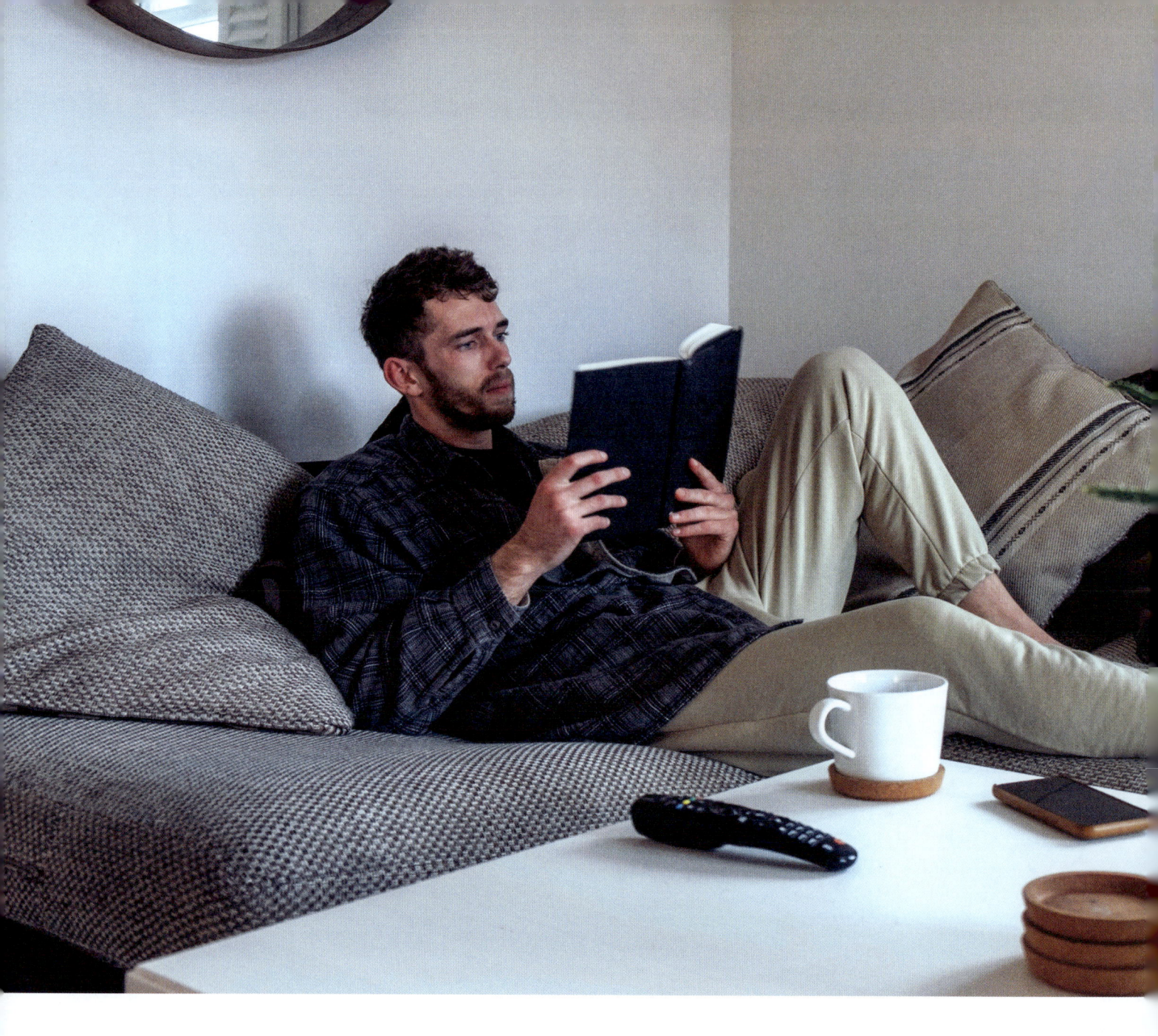

Above: Make time to get stuck into a good book, if that's what brings you joy

WHAT DO WE MEAN BY 'WORK'?

First, it's important to define what we mean by work. Commonly, we mean a paid job, where we have to show up for a set number of hours on a set number of days. But when it comes to a work-life balance, it's not the case that work is 'work' and everything else is 'life'.

If you are in a paid working role, then your work time includes all your time spent commuting, overtime and any time spent answering emails or calls outside of your core hours. If you're catching up on projects in the evenings, or logging in at weekends, it's all work.

Work also includes any other commitments and responsibilities in your daily life. You may have a caring role, whether that's as a parent, or for a parent. This could include things like transporting family members to classes or events, personal care, supervision, preparing meals and so on. Work also includes household tasks, like chores and cooking, and life admin, such as bill paying and taking the car to the garage.

Work, in this context, is anything that is essential to the daily running of your home life and work life. These are things that you generally don't engage with purely for fun or personal enjoyment, but that are required as part of your life. Of course, work and life can overlap – spending time with your children, if you have any, for example, can consist of both essential 'work' tasks and enjoyable 'life' tasks.

WHAT CONSTITUTES THE 'LIFE' PART?

The other side of this coin is 'life'. This is where you do things that you enjoy, because you want to and not just because you have to. So this might include things like hobbies and interests (we focus on these in more detail on pages 48-53), and making sure you include time to do these.

Life might also include exercise and recreation. Not everyone enjoys exercise, and it can feel like work, but if you find an activity you enjoy, you can get the benefits of being physically fit and healthy while also having fun.

Then there is time spent with other people. This might be quality time with your family, going on day trips, or simply relaxing playing a game and watching a film. It's also time spent socialising with your friends. Connecting with other people outside of work is important for our social health, and to help us relax and switch off from the work side of life.

Life can also include spending time alone, doing a solo hobby and enjoying some downtime. That could be reading, playing video games, working on a collection or creating something, or catching up on the latest Netflix series.

Generally, things in the 'life' bracket are those things that you choose to do because you want to. It's important to note that sleep is a very important part of a work-life balance that doesn't really fit into either category. It's essential to our mental and physical health, and a good, balanced life will include the right amount of sleep for you; too little

A mindful work-life balance

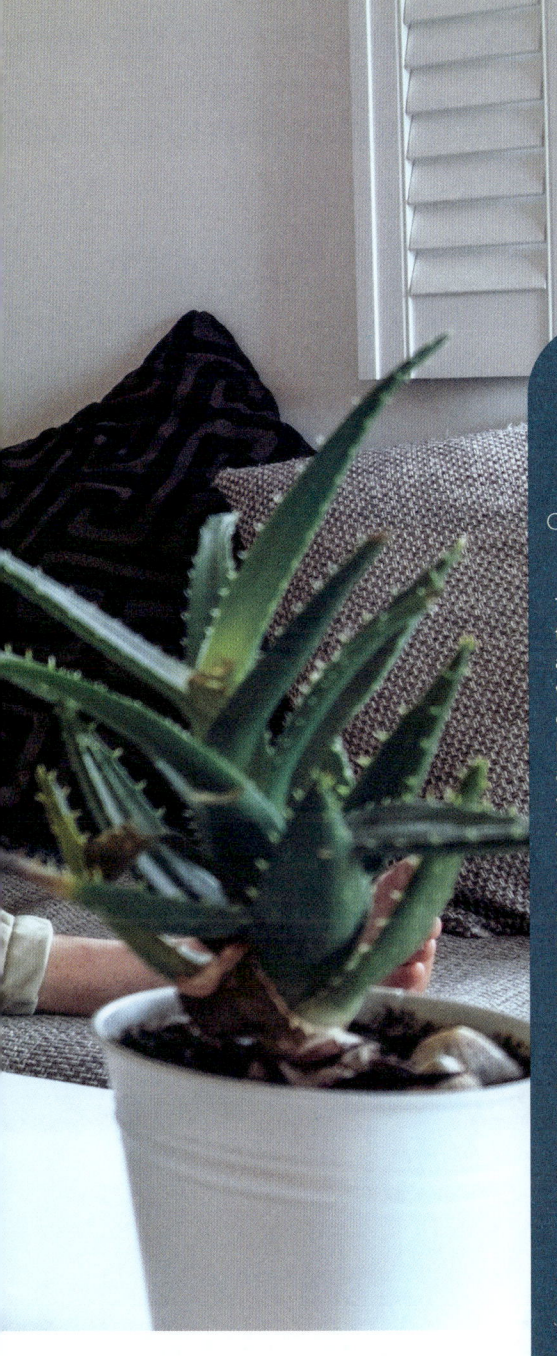

Common obstacles and how to overcome them
Common pitfalls to avoid on your way to finding a work-life balance

There are plenty of things that can prevent you from achieving your perfect work-life balance. Some of these are, by necessity, unavoidable. But there are other obstacles that you can overcome. For a start, many of us are too hard on ourselves and will admit to being a bit of a perfectionist. While this can be a good quality, sometimes 'good enough' is okay to free up time for other areas of your life. In this modern world, we're also very accessible all the time with smartphones and social media. Try to set aside times when you're not available, so you can focus on other things in your life more mindfully – if you're with family or friends, switch off your notifications and just enjoy being in the moment. It's okay if you don't respond to a message immediately (unless it's truly urgent). Reply when the time is right for you to engage properly with the subject at hand. If you practise mindfulness in life, you can aim to be truly present in what you're doing in the here and now, rather than feeling all areas of your life colliding into one.

and it can be very hard to maintain that work-life balance.

YOUR CURRENT WORK-LIFE BALANCE
Now you have an understanding of what we mean by a work-life balance, it's time to have a good look at your current balance. We have some activities to help you with this, encouraging you to think about how you spend your typical day right now and what you would like your typical day to look like.

We can't often achieve our perfect work-life balance. We're sure many of you would love to work less and play more, but there are often unavoidable factors to consider. You might be contracted to work a certain number of hours per week, or you may have all-day caring responsibilities at home so that a partner can go to work, for example. These are just a couple of scenarios – no two lives are the same, and what a work-life balance looks like for you will be completely different to someone else's.

My typical day

Pick a selection of colours to represent paid work (including time spent commuting), family work, household chores, life admin, leisure time, exercise time and sleep time. Colour in the average blocks of time you spend on each of these to see what your current work-life balance looks like.

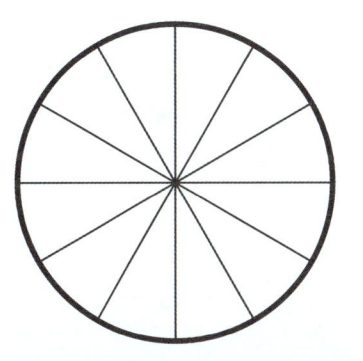

WORKING FROM HOME
If you work from home, the boundaries can become more blurred. Make sure you stick to a routine.

Mindfulness for Men

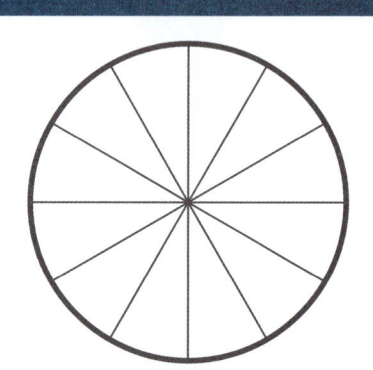

My goal day

Now complete the same activity as on the previous page, but this time colour in the average blocks of time you would like to spend on each of these in the future. It's important to be realistic – some segments are fixed (i.e. work patterns or family commitments) – but think about what you would like to achieve with the rest of your time.

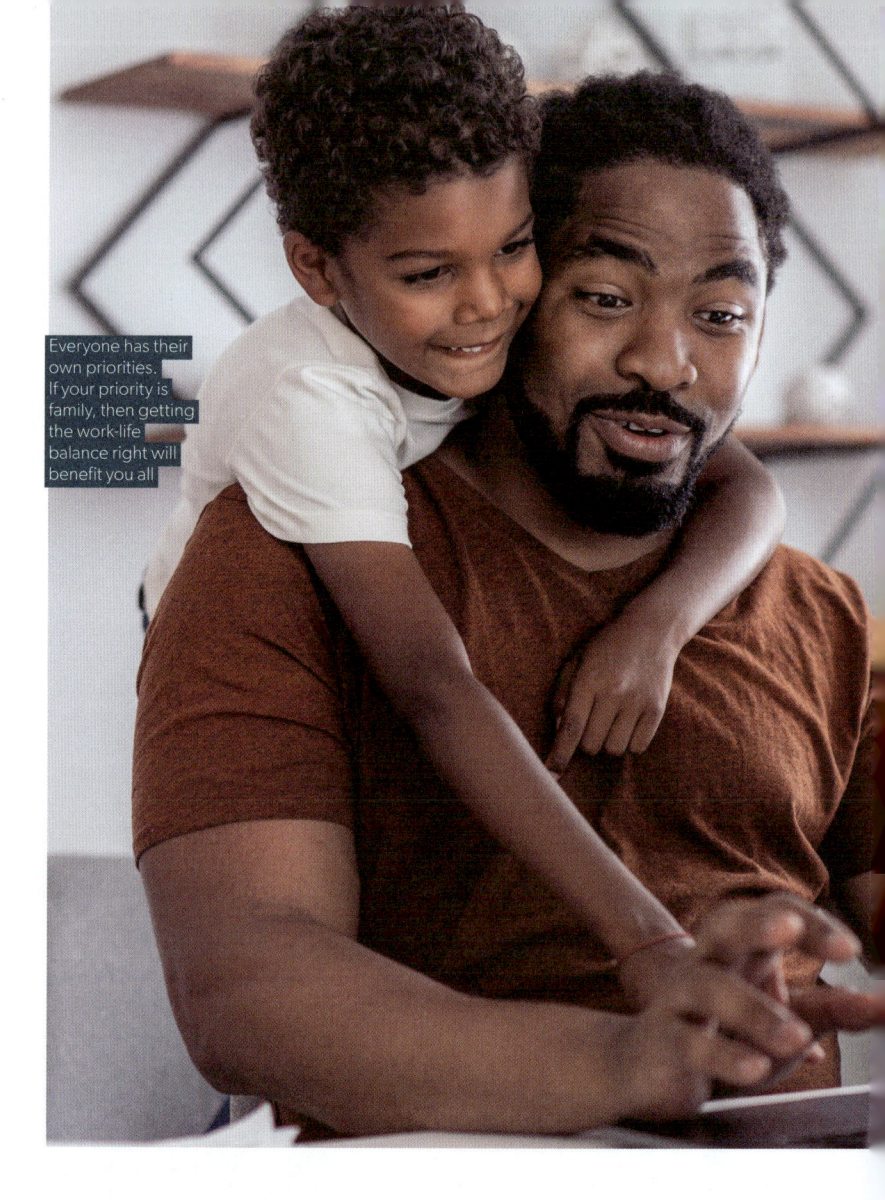

Everyone has their own priorities. If your priority is family, then getting the work-life balance right will benefit you all

However, what you can do is look at the time you have outside of your work commitments. Are you using it wisely? Do you have a window in your day when you could fit in some exercise to give you an energy boost, or do you want a chance to read or play a game to relax in the evening? Try to think about what you want to achieve in your weekly schedule and compare that to what your schedule looks like now.

WORKING TOWARDS YOUR GOAL
Of course, there will inevitably have to be a measure of compromise, especially if you're in a family household with shared responsibilities. But even making small steps towards a better work-life balance can make a huge difference.

The first thing to do is to be more mindful around your work-life balance. It can be so easy to get caught up in the day-to-day that we don't stop to consider whether it's really working for us. Every so often, take a step back and really think about your work-life balance, see what improvements you can make, and then set yourself a reminder to audit your life again in three months or six months. You might find that your improvements are having a positive impact, or you might find that you have slipped back into old habits. The key is being aware of this and taking action before you start to feel the repercussions of an unbalanced life.

There will be obstacles that are in your way – some are caused by other

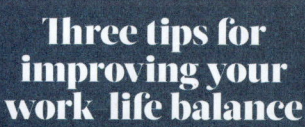

Three tips for improving your work-life balance
These are the three key areas to focus on to improve your work-life balance

1

SEPARATE WORK FROM HOME
If you work outside the home, this is a bit easier. Try not to bring work documents home with you, and be strict about when you answer calls or reply to emails. If you work from home, try to have a designated workspace. If it's a shared common space, like the dining table, set up and clear away your work stuff to signal the beginning and end of your working day.

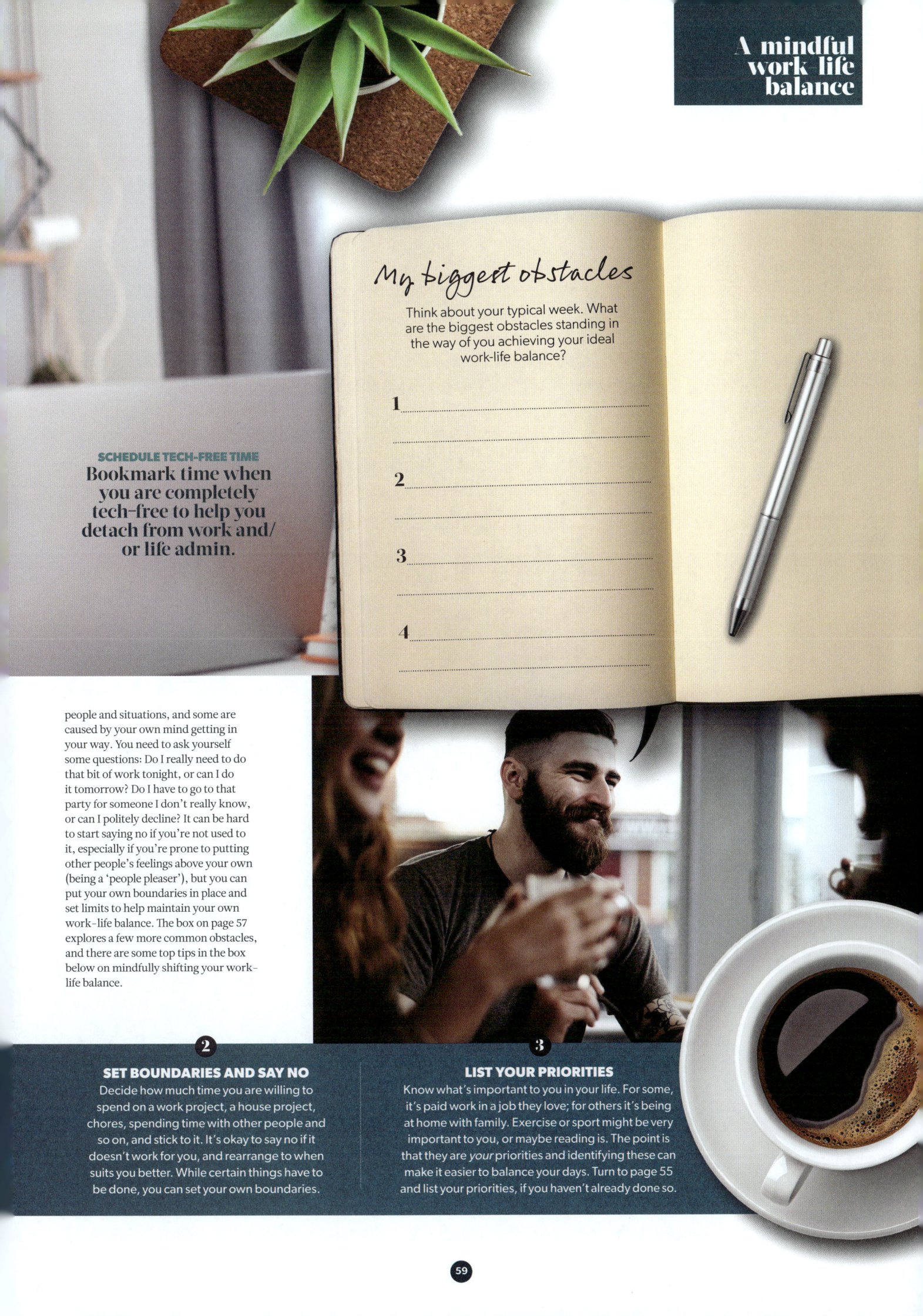

A mindful work-life balance

My biggest obstacles

Think about your typical week. What are the biggest obstacles standing in the way of you achieving your ideal work-life balance?

1. ....
2. ....
3. ....
4. ....

SCHEDULE TECH-FREE TIME
Bookmark time when you are completely tech-free to help you detach from work and/or life admin.

people and situations, and some are caused by your own mind getting in your way. You need to ask yourself some questions: Do I really need to do that bit of work tonight, or can I do it tomorrow? Do I have to go to that party for someone I don't really know, or can I politely decline? It can be hard to start saying no if you're not used to it, especially if you're prone to putting other people's feelings above your own (being a 'people pleaser'), but you can put your own boundaries in place and set limits to help maintain your own work-life balance. The box on page 57 explores a few more common obstacles, and there are some top tips in the box below on mindfully shifting your work-life balance.

2
SET BOUNDARIES AND SAY NO
Decide how much time you are willing to spend on a work project, a house project, chores, spending time with other people and so on, and stick to it. It's okay to say no if it doesn't work for you, and rearrange to when suits you better. While certain things have to be done, you can set your own boundaries.

3
LIST YOUR PRIORITIES
Know what's important to you in your life. For some, it's paid work in a job they love; for others it's being at home with family. Exercise or sport might be very important to you, or maybe reading is. The point is that they are *your* priorities and identifying these can make it easier to balance your days. Turn to page 55 and list your priorities, if you haven't already done so.

Mindfulness for Men

We explore how to be mindful about your mental health and when you might need extra help

UNDERSTANDING MENTAL HEALTH

YOU'RE NOT ALONE
One in eight adult men have a common mental health problem, statistics from the Mental Health Foundation show.

Disabilities and mental health

Physical and developmental disabilities can impact on your mental health and the chance of experiencing some mental health conditions

If you have a disability, you might be more likely to experience some mental health conditions. This can include physical disabilities, as well as developmental disabilities such as autism or ADHD. Sometimes, living with a disability can make daily life more difficult in some areas, which can lead to feelings of frustration, or situations might be more stressful. Those with a developmental disability that impacts on social situations and relationships, as well as a difficulty in managing feelings, may be more likely to experience depression and anxiety. If you live with a disability, then it can be even more important to be mindful about your mental health and seek support if you are feeling worried or stressed. Speak to your doctor or specialist, and they can refer you to relevant support and resources.

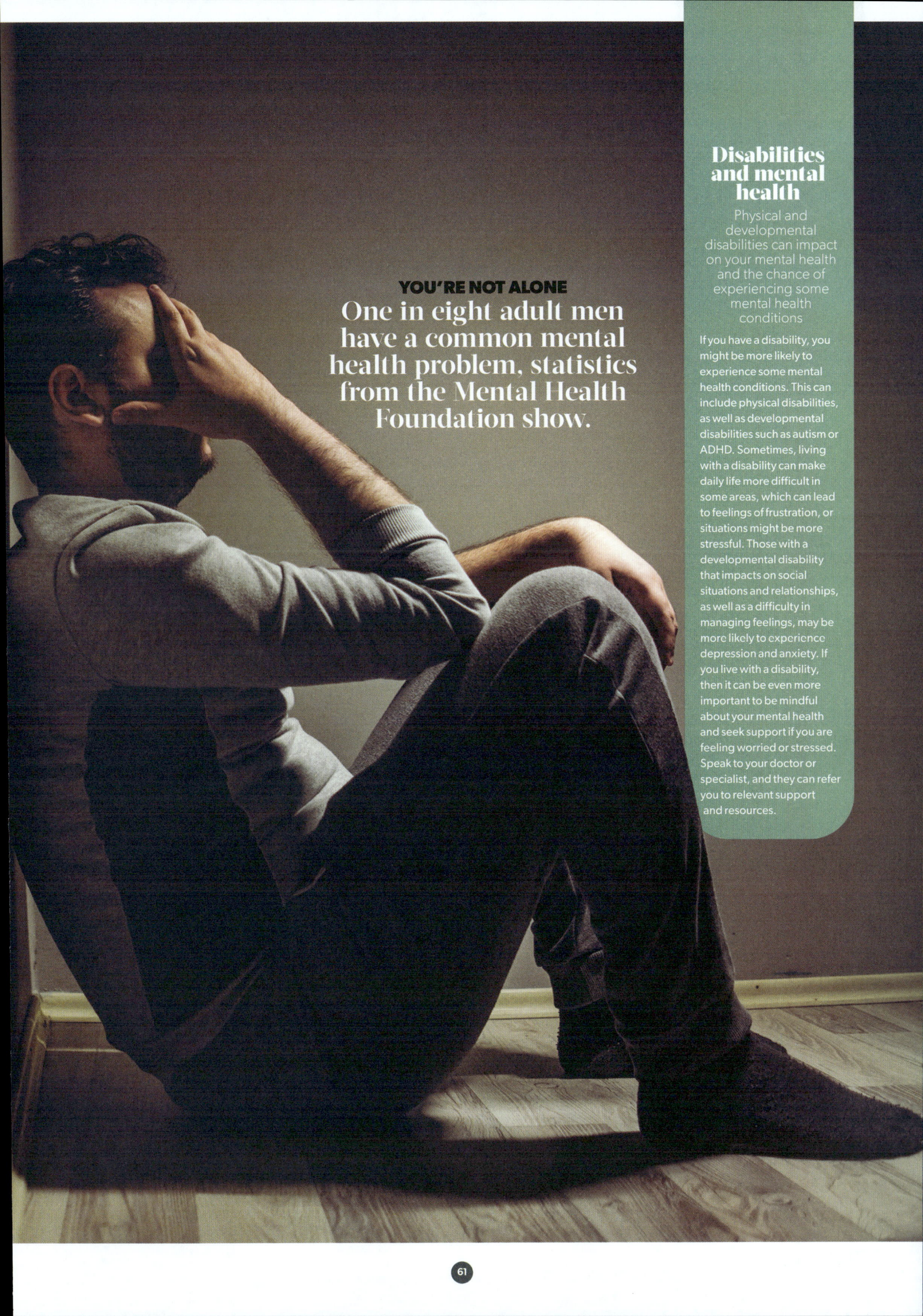

Mindfulness for Men

Mental health can be a difficult topic to talk about and think about, but it's just as important as physical health. Just as we need to be mindful about what's going on in our bodies, we also need to develop an awareness of our state of mind if we want to achieve optimum health and wellbeing.

You could be reading this from any number of situations – maybe you haven't really considered your mental health too much before; maybe you have experienced a mental health problem either in the past or at the present time; or maybe you have noticed some changes in your mental health, but you're not sure how to manage them. What we're encouraging you to do in this feature is explore your current mental health, put in place tools and coping strategies for good mental health, and then look at how to remain mindful of your mental health long-term.

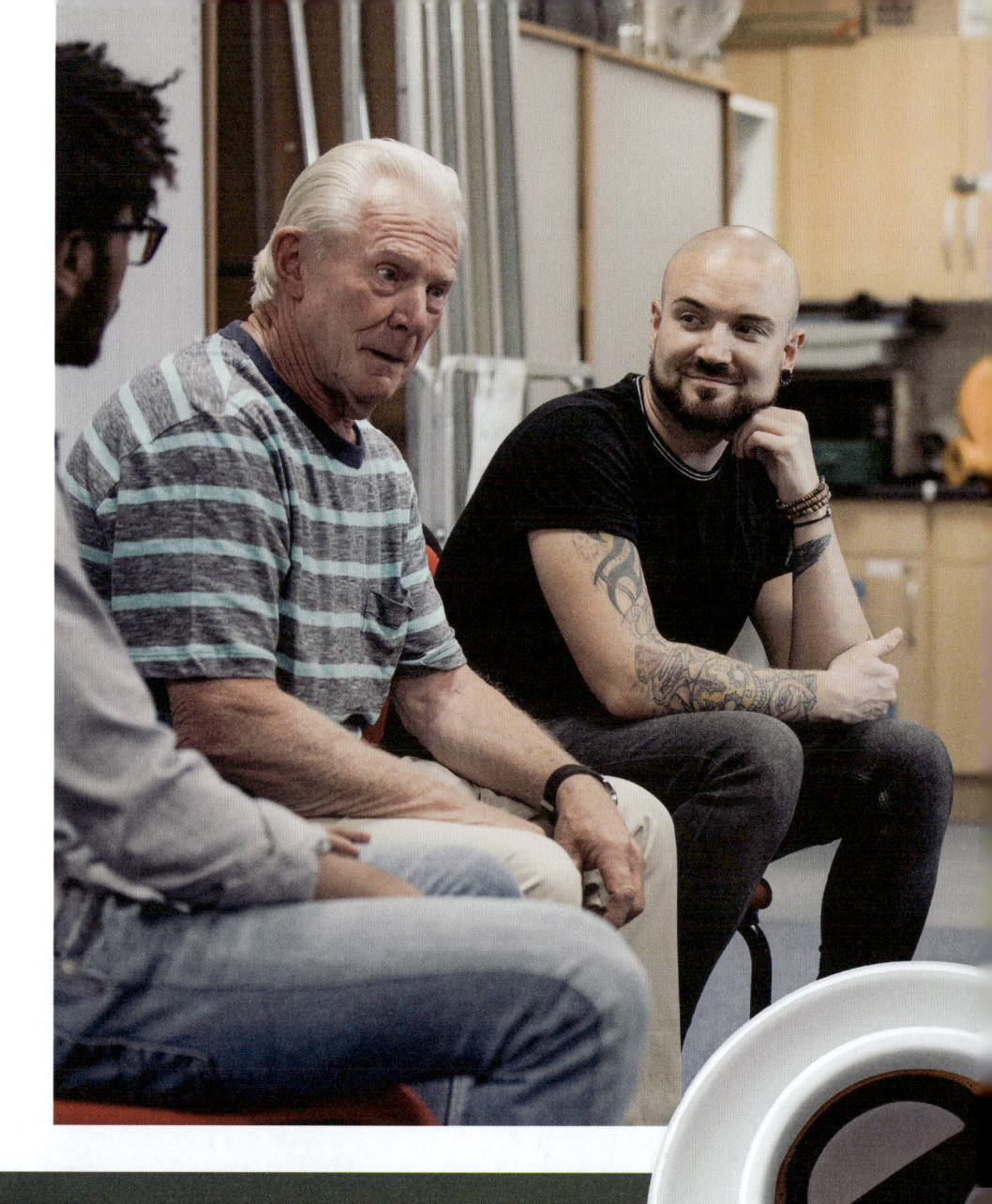

Self-care toolkit

Think of a time when you have felt anxious, worried, stressed or sad. Then try to think of things that you can do to help ease those emotions. Here you can write down anything that helps to create a self-care toolkit you can refer to when you need a mental health boost. Fill in each section with a specific emotion, such as 'stressed', and something you can do to help, such as 'go for a walk'.

WHEN I FEEL ....

I KNOW IT HELPS ME TO ....

WHEN I FEEL ....

I KNOW IT HELPS ME TO ....

WHEN I FEEL ....

I KNOW IT HELPS ME TO ....

My worries and concerns

Use this space to write down any specific worries and concerns that you are experiencing in your life right now. It doesn't matter whether it's something big or a small concern; it's important to address any worries you may have.

....
....
....
....
....
....
....
....
....

Asking for help

If you're worried about your mental health, then it's time to ask for help

Understanding mental health

WHAT DO WE MEAN BY MENTAL HEALTH?

Your mental health refers to your emotional, psychological and social wellbeing, and affects the way that you think, feel, act and respond to external stresses. When you have good mental health, it means that you think and feel in a way that enables you to be able to live the life that you want. Your mental health can also influence your behaviours, perceptions and cognition, which can then affect external things like your relationships, ability to cope under stress, decision-making skills, and how you react to the world around you. It's about how well you can regulate your feelings and emotions.

That's quite a broad range of things, which is why our mental health is so important. Mental health and physical health are two sides of the same coin, and therefore need to be given the same priority in our lives. The two often interact – when you're in a state of poor mental health, you might feel bad physically too, and find it difficult to motivate yourself to do the things you need to look after your physical body. If you neglect your physical health, you may then find that your mental health starts to decline. If you're going through a busy period at work, for example, you might not find the time to exercise, eat well and get enough sleep, which can lead to poorer mental health outcomes.

Our mental health ebbs and flows throughout our life, and that's normal. You can't expect to feel good all of the time. You will have days when you feel a little low, tired or rundown. If you notice this happening, you can start to do something about it, taking extra rest or spending some time outside in nature.

However, sometimes, poor mental health can mean that we experience mental health conditions. This can be overwhelming and quite scary, especially if you've never experienced a mental health problem before. We'll explore some of the most common mental health problems further on in this feature.

MENTAL HEALTH IN MEN

While mental health problems can happen to any of us at any time, there are some differences between men's and women's experiences. Some of these are symptomatic – for example, while depression is the same condition in both men and women, some symptoms are more common in men. According to the Mental Health Foundation in the UK, this includes irritability, anger, loss of control, risk taking and aggression. Men are also more likely to look for external coping solutions, such as an increased dependence on alcohol or drugs, for example, or taking on extra work as a distraction from other issues. Men are

Above: Asking for help can be difficult, but talking about how you're feeling is a great way to improve your mental health

MY MENTAL HEALTH

How do you feel about your mental health right now? Do you have any concerns or worries, or do you feel you have good mental health? Use the scale to circle how concerned you are about your mental health right now.

NOT CONCERNED

1

2

3

4

5

VERY CONCERNED

*Please note, if you're concerned or very concerned about your mental health, you should seek help from a professional source.

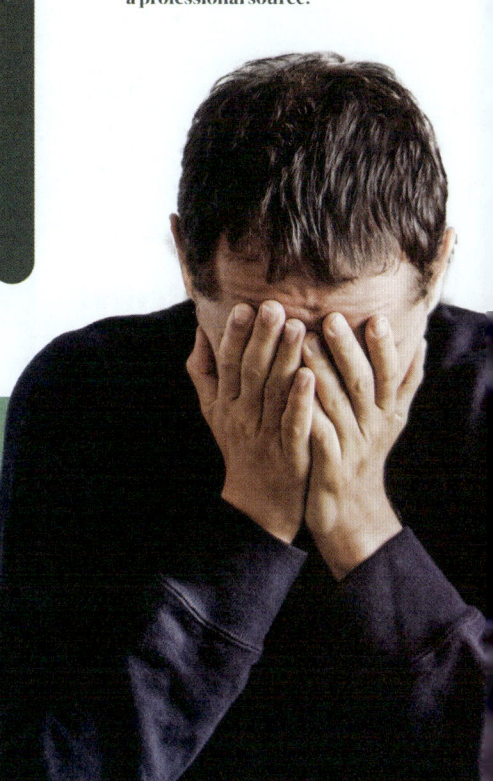

It can be hard to ask for help, especially if you're not used to talking about how you're feeling. We have a feature on talking on pages 68-69, but it's particularly important to seek help if you're worried about your mental health. It's best to seek support early on when you first notice that you are experiencing low mental health. This enables you to access resources more quickly and start to put tools in place. You don't have to have a specific mental health condition to ask for help. You may feel that you're finding it hard to enjoy life, you're having thoughts or feelings that you're struggling with, you're more stressed than usual, you're not sleeping well and/or you're feeling low on energy. If you can, book a doctor's appointment and explain how you're feeling; this will help them to direct you to the best help for you. This might be talking therapies, medication or a referral to local support services.

Mindfulness for Men

Gratitude

Regularly practising gratitude has been shown to have a positive effect on mental health and wellbeing. It enables you to mindfully review your day and think about those things you are grateful for. These can be the people around you or physical things like a warm house. Or it can be little things that have happened in your day to make you feel happy. Try to keep track for the next few days and see how you feel.

Date	Things I am grateful for today
Date	Things I am grateful for today
Date	Things I am grateful for today

Emergency contact list

Write down a list of contact details that you can use if you are worried about your mental health. This might include your doctor, a support helpline or someone you trust.

Name	Contact details
Name	Contact details
Name	Contact details

PRACTISE GRATITUDE
Regularly considering things you're grateful for can boost your mental health (try the activity above to get started).

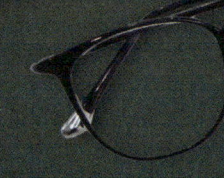

also less likely to access therapy than women (one statistic from the NHS in the UK shows that only 38% of all referrals to talking therapies are for men).

However, the tools, techniques and therapies that are available work equally well across both sexes. Sadly, archaic and unhelpful societal pressures can contribute to the reason why men are less likely to talk about their mental health and to access the help they need. We live in a world where, for a very long time, a construct of gender stereotypes has been built up. This isn't helped by the portrayal of men in the media or on television – always strong, resilient, dependable, never showing weakness or taking time for self-care. While some of these attributes are good – there's nothing wrong with being strong and resilient – it's also important to learn to embrace all emotions, and be mindful of our mental health and the things we need to do to protect it.

There are some signs of the tide turning away from these old-fashioned views of masculinity. In recent years, there have been numerous campaigns to encourage men to talk more about how they are feeling (again, refer to pages 68-69 for more on talking) and to be more open about any mental health issues they might be experiencing. If you grew up in a time when you heard a lot of 'man up' and 'don't cry' type phrases, then there is a lot of unpicking to do to become comfortable in showing emotion. This often starts with asking for help, or being honest with a loved one. It's also about not being afraid to cry, the body's normal and healthy physical reaction to an emotional state or pain.

This can be very hard if you feel that there is a stigma against this, which might have started from your very early days at school. However, we hope that these perceptions will be abolished in

Mental health resources

Here are five apps and websites you can use to help manage your mental health every day

❶ ACTION FOR HAPPINESS
ACTIONFORHAPPINESS.ORG / IOS AND ANDROID; FREE

Action for Happiness is available online or as an app, and is packed with tips, tools and resources to help you live a happier life. There are monthly challenges you can take part in, or you can connect with like-minded individuals. It looks at things you can do to make yourself happier, but also how to make others around you happier too.

❷ MOODKIT
IOS ONLY; ONE-OFF PAYMENT APPLIES

This app has received a lot of praise in both the UK and the USA as a great mental health app. It helps you to apply the strategies of professional psychology in your own life, through four integrated tools. It uses the principles of CBT, with more than 200 mood-improvement activities.

Understanding mental health

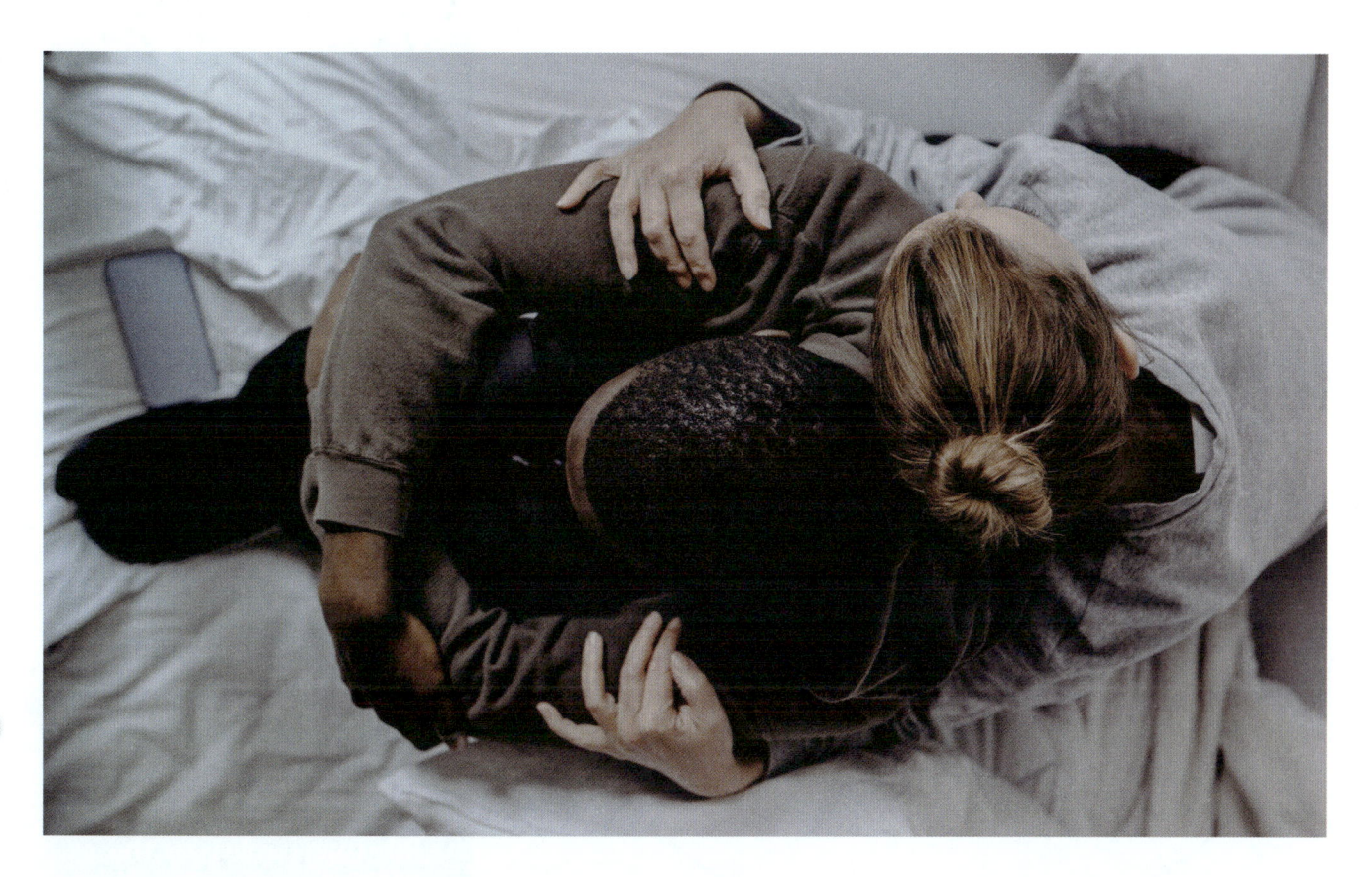

time, and that men's mental health can be talked about openly, honestly and thoughtfully in all areas of society.

MENTAL HEALTH PROBLEMS
How do you know if you're in a temporary period of poorer mental health, or suffering from a mental health problem? There are usually some initial signs, which often begin with changes in your mood, difficulty enjoying life in the way you usually do, feelings of stress, and problems with sleeping, which continue over many days, weeks or months.

There are many types of mental health problems that you might experience. Depression is one of the most common, which is a low mood that lasts a long time and impacts on your day-to-day life. You may feel like you don't want to do anything, that it's all a bit hopeless. This can be mild, where you can cope with daily tasks but everything feels hard, or far more severe. It can, in advanced cases, be life-threatening. This is why it's important to be aware of the signs of depression and seek help early on.

Another common mental health problem is anxiety, which is an ongoing feeling of worry or fear above and beyond a normal anxiety response. This can even manifest in physical symptoms, such as headaches or difficulty breathing. You may even experience panic attacks, a natural fear response but very unsettling to go through. Anxiety can be treated with CBT (cognitive behaviour therapy) type therapies, where you learn to change the way you think and behave in certain situations.

Mental health problems can be triggered as a result of particular circumstances. For example, if you have a lot going on all at one time, you might find that your stress levels increase. It's normal to feel a little stress from time to time, but a lot of stress over a longer period of time can really impact on your mental health (and your physical health too). You may also experience mental health problems as a result of a specific trauma or when bereaved – these circumstances can lead to a period of low mental health, understandably, and can take a little time and support to recover from.

3
BETTERHELP – THERAPY
BETTERHELP.COM / IOS AND ANDROID; REGULAR FEE APPLIES
This is not the cheapest solution, but if you want to access a therapist through digital means, this is a good option. You get matched with a therapist who you can talk to and work through issues with. This can work for you if you're unsure about meeting with a therapist in person, or if waiting lists are long in your area.

1
MENTAL HEALTH FOUNDATION (UK)
MENTALHEALTH.ORG.UK
This website has lots of handy resources you can access, as well as information specifically around men's mental health. If you're looking for tips, advice and support, then this is a good place to start.

5
IBREATHE – RELAX AND BREATHE
IOS ONLY; FREE, WITH OPTIONAL IN-APP PURCHASE TO REMOVE ADS
This simple app guides you through deep breathing exercises and breathwork when you need help to calm down or lower your stress levels. This includes things like box breathing and 4-7-8 breathing. It also integrates with Apple Health, and has an Apple Watch app.

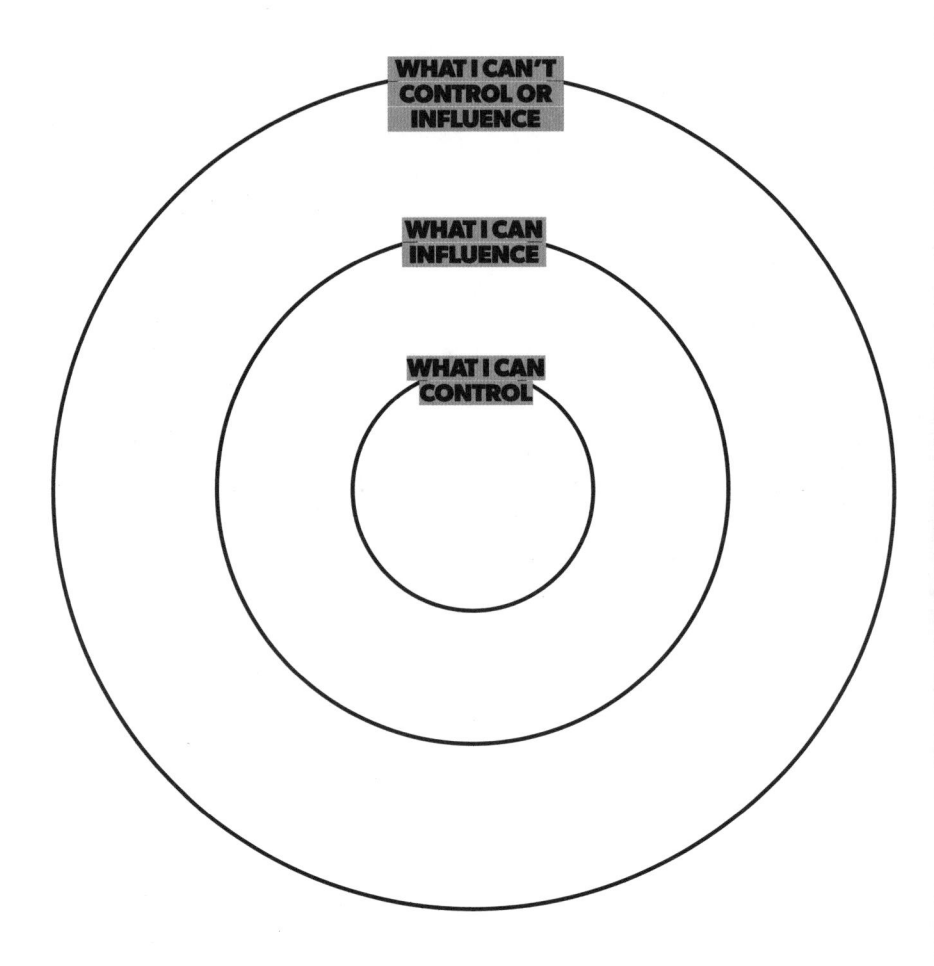

Mindfulness for Men

[Diagram: Three concentric circles labeled from outer to inner: "WHAT I CAN'T CONTROL OR INFLUENCE", "WHAT I CAN INFLUENCE", "WHAT I CAN CONTROL"]

WHAT I CAN CONTROL

Thinking about your worries and concerns, try this exercise. The inside circle represents everything that you can control directly yourself, so this might be things like limiting time on social media, regular exercise and so on.

Then, the middle circle is those things you can influence, which might be things like your relationships and friendships.

The final circle is for those things that you have no control or influence over, such as large world events. This exercise can help you put worries and concerns into perspective, and enable you to only focus on those things you can control or influence.

There are many other mental health conditions that manifest in different ways and impact on your life with different levels of severity. This is why mindfulness around mental health is so important – you need to know what your 'normal' is, so you can be more attuned to when you feel something is off. This helps you to identify any mental health issues earlier and seek the help you need, or put into practice any tools and techniques you know help you.

BEING MINDFUL AROUND MENTAL HEALTH

There are a few ways that you can become more mindful of your mental health. Keeping a journal can be a useful exercise. If you've never done it before, it can feel too much to write huge paragraphs every day, but there are other options. You could simply keep a mood journal, where you pick a colour for different moods and colour each day so that you can visually see any patterns. Or you could write short bullet points into a notes app on your phone. The more you tune in to your mental health and write down how you're feeling day to day, the more natural it will feel.

If you do notice that you are struggling with your mental health, then there are things you can do. If you feel a little stressed, tired, overwhelmed or sad, then many of the things that we talk about in this book can really help. Meditation can help to bring calmness to your mind and help you to explore some of your thoughts and feelings. You can also use the relaxation feature (pages 70-75) to help you find some peace, or indulge in one of your hobbies and interests (pages 48-53) to lift your mood.

Exercise is just as important to our mental health as it is our physical health (see pages 76-81), so it's worth making time to move. If you can do it outside, even better, as we know that being outside in the fresh air is good for our mental health. It's important to sleep well (see pages 92-95), and to see friends and family (see pages 20-25 and 26-29).

However, if none of these strategies are working for you, then it's time to look for more professional help and advice. There is no shame in seeking help for a mental health condition; you wouldn't walk around with a broken leg trying to get on with your life as normal, so don't ignore a problem with your mental health either. The sooner you address the way you are feeling, the sooner you can get the right support and start your journey back to good mental health once again.

Understanding mental health

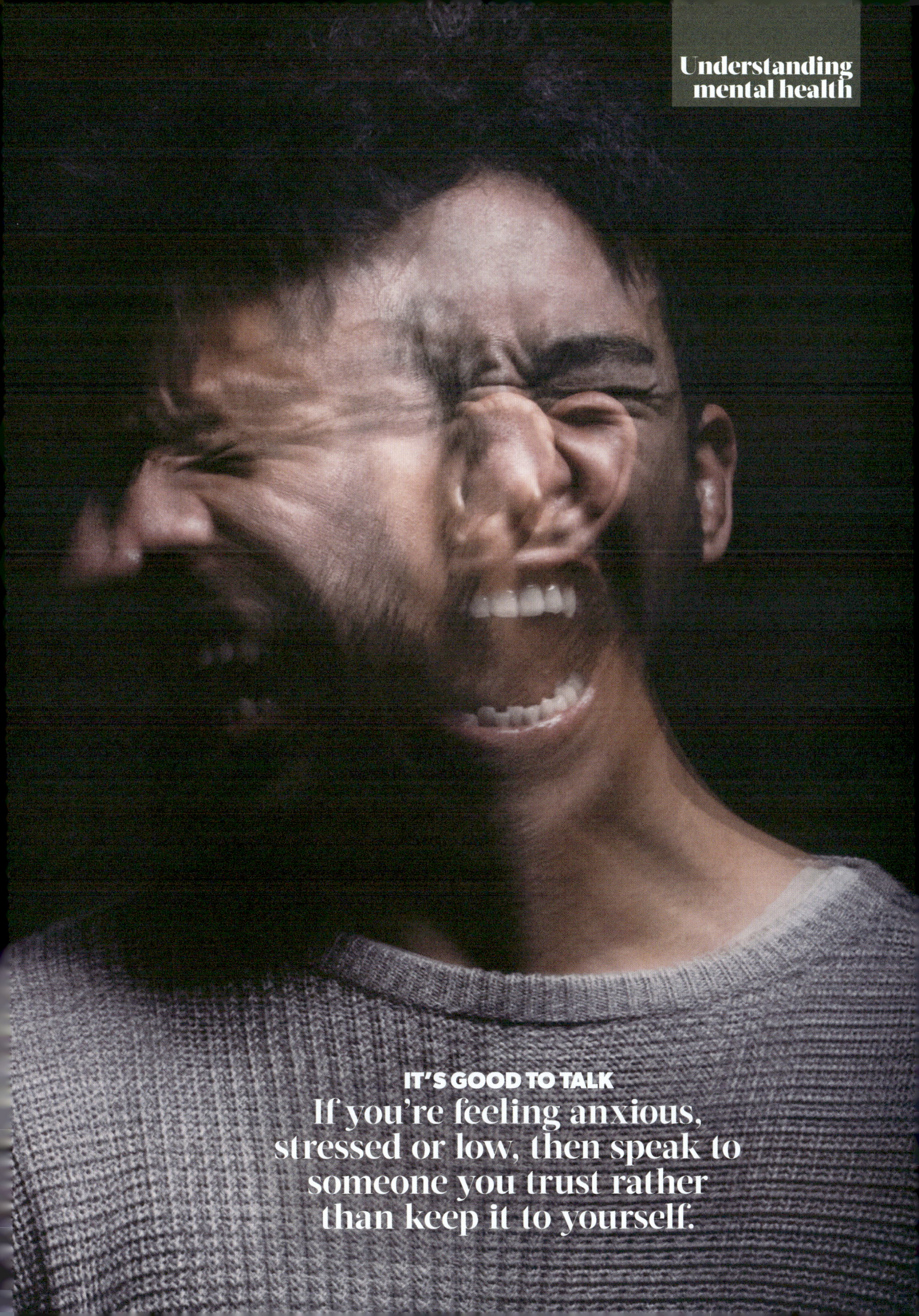

IT'S GOOD TO TALK
If you're feeling anxious, stressed or low, then speak to someone you trust rather than keep it to yourself.

Mindfulness for Men

WHY IT'S IMPORTANT TO TALK

Talking doesn't always come naturally, but it can help to improve your wellbeing and mental health

Talking is an important part of life. It helps us to build connections and foster strong relationships, to communicate at work, and to share hobbies and interests. It can be hard, however, to talk about things like emotions, feelings, worries and concerns. Internalising these thoughts can make it harder to confront them and solve our issues, which can build up and contribute towards higher stress levels, mental health conditions like depression and anxiety, and even some physical symptoms such as headaches and pain.

Men often find it harder than women to talk to others about these kinds of thoughts and feelings. There are many reasons for this, some of which are societal and some are physiological.

My contact list
Use this space to write down the people in your life you feel you could talk to if you need to, so you can refer back to it in the future.

Name ....
Address ....
Email ....
Phone ....

Name ....
Address ....
Email ....
Phone ....

Name ....
Address ....
Email ....
Phone ....

Name ....
Address ....
Email ....
Phone ....

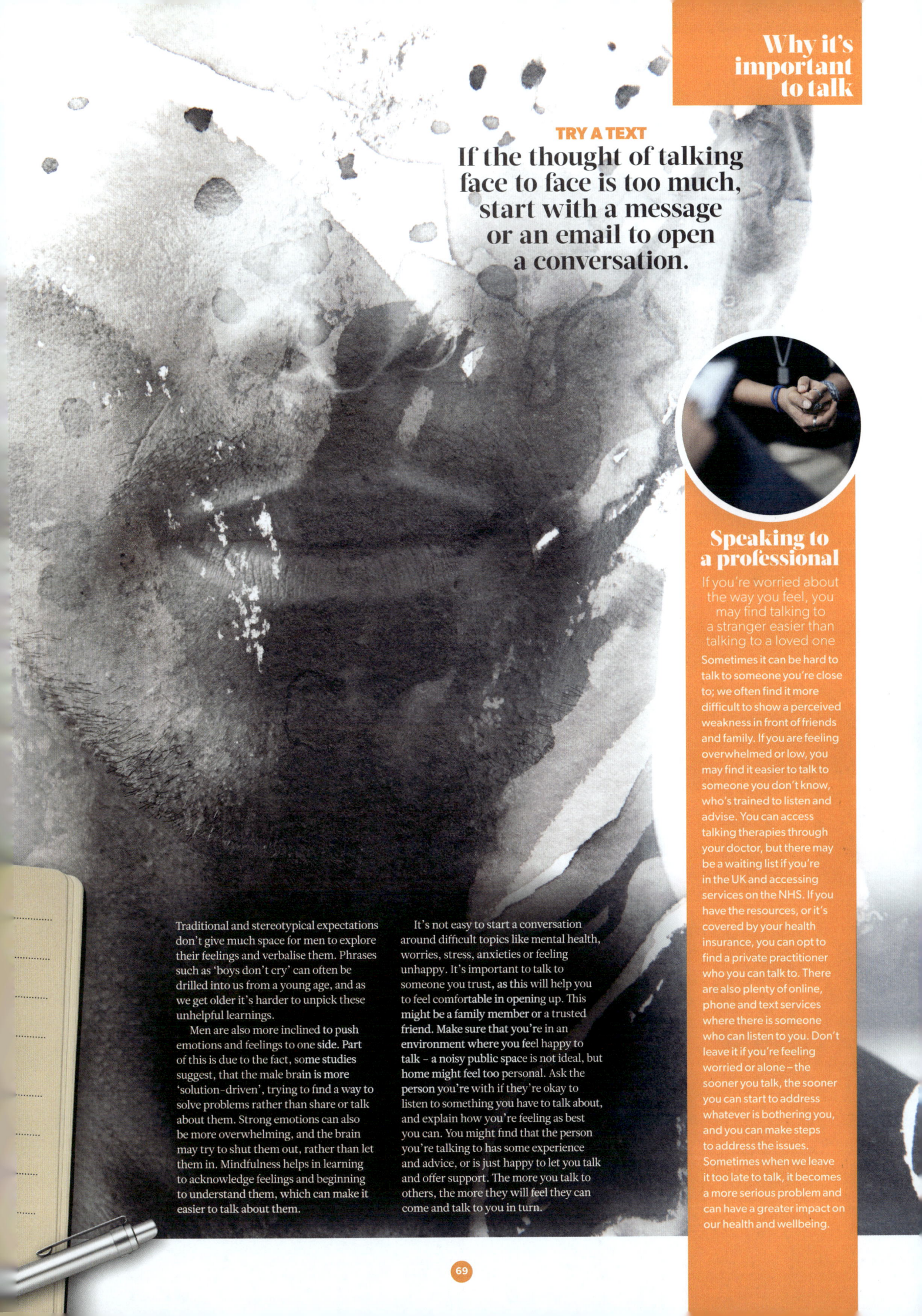

Why it's important to talk

TRY A TEXT

If the thought of talking face to face is too much, start with a message or an email to open a conversation.

Speaking to a professional

If you're worried about the way you feel, you may find talking to a stranger easier than talking to a loved one

Sometimes it can be hard to talk to someone you're close to; we often find it more difficult to show a perceived weakness in front of friends and family. If you are feeling overwhelmed or low, you may find it easier to talk to someone you don't know, who's trained to listen and advise. You can access talking therapies through your doctor, but there may be a waiting list if you're in the UK and accessing services on the NHS. If you have the resources, or it's covered by your health insurance, you can opt to find a private practitioner who you can talk to. There are also plenty of online, phone and text services where there is someone who can listen to you. Don't leave it if you're feeling worried or alone – the sooner you talk, the sooner you can start to address whatever is bothering you, and you can make steps to address the issues. Sometimes when we leave it too late to talk, it becomes a more serious problem and can have a greater impact on our health and wellbeing.

Traditional and stereotypical expectations don't give much space for men to explore their feelings and verbalise them. Phrases such as 'boys don't cry' can often be drilled into us from a young age, and as we get older it's harder to unpick these unhelpful learnings.

Men are also more inclined to push emotions and feelings to one side. Part of this is due to the fact, some studies suggest, that the male brain is more 'solution-driven', trying to find a way to solve problems rather than share or talk about them. Strong emotions can also be more overwhelming, and the brain may try to shut them out, rather than let them in. Mindfulness helps in learning to acknowledge feelings and beginning to understand them, which can make it easier to talk about them.

It's not easy to start a conversation around difficult topics like mental health, worries, stress, anxieties or feeling unhappy. It's important to talk to someone you trust, as this will help you to feel comfortable in opening up. This might be a family member or a trusted friend. Make sure that you're in an environment where you feel happy to talk – a noisy public space is not ideal, but home might feel too personal. Ask the person you're with if they're okay to listen to something you have to talk about, and explain how you're feeling as best you can. You might find that the person you're talking to has some experience and advice, or is just happy to let you talk and offer support. The more you talk to others, the more they will feel they can come and talk to you in turn.

Mindfulness for Men

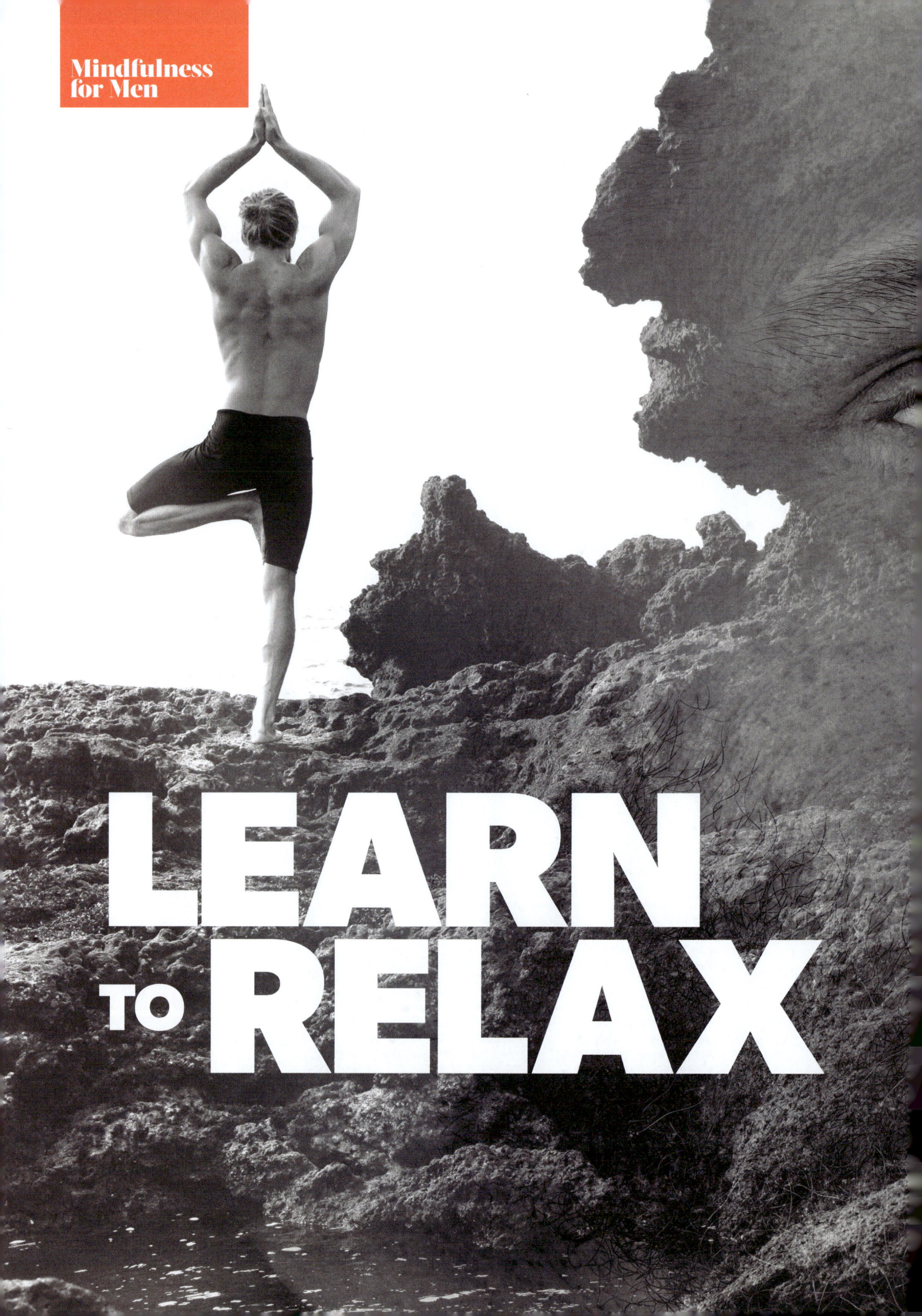

LEARN TO RELAX

Learn to relax

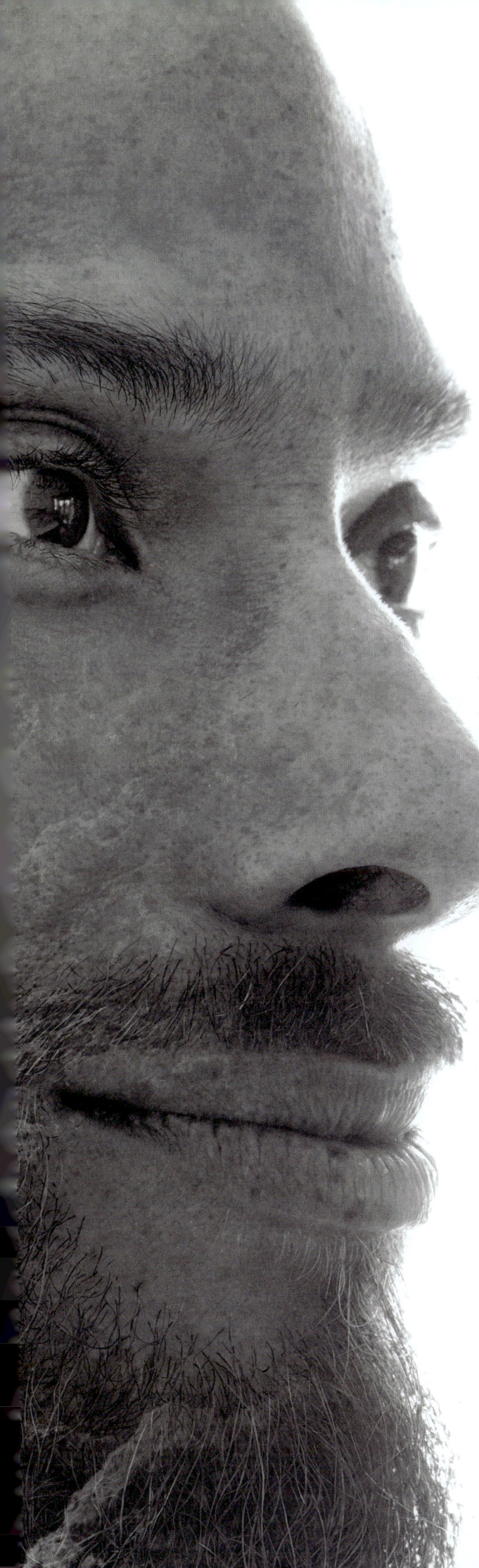

Relaxation doesn't come naturally to all of us, but being more mindful about it can help improve your mindset

How much thought do you give to relaxation? Chances are that it's not enough. Are you someone who goes on a holiday and suddenly feels relaxed for the first time in months? It's not uncommon for us to live our lives so fast and busy that we forget to relax until we're forced to, whether that's by a planned holiday or an unfortunate event such as illness or injury.

Relaxation is a key part of life, and not something that should be an afterthought. Rather than only considering relaxing once or twice a year, you should be incorporating relaxation into your daily life. If you spend a lot of your life being busy, stressed or worried, then relaxing can help give you a break, both physically and mentally. It's not going to eliminate the cause of your stress or anxiety, but it can help you reset and cope better with situations.

There are lots of different ways that you can relax, which may overlap with some of your personal hobbies (see pages 48-53 for more on hobbies and interests). A relaxing activity should be something that truly helps you to switch off, wind down and feel calm. In this section, we'll be exploring how you can be more mindful about your relaxation, and give you some advice on how to incorporate it into your life.

WHY DO WE NEED TO RELAX?

It's really important to note that relaxation isn't 'being lazy'. It's absolutely essential to your wellbeing to find some time to switch off. The time when you're asleep doesn't count – we're talking about active relaxation in your waking hours. Many people do choose to do something relaxing in the hours before bed, as this can help them sleep, whereas others prefer to start their day with relaxation before the busyness begins.

Relaxing properly has an impact on your mind and body. Mentally, when you relax and switch off, it gives your mind a break from everything else going on around you. It helps to reduce anxiety and relieve stress. Regular relaxation can also help to protect against certain mental health conditions, such as depression.

When we're in busy or intense situations, our body triggers a stress response. This makes your heart rate speed up, your muscles may feel tense, you might experience headaches, and your emotions could be a bit up and down. While being in that stress response state isn't going to do much harm short term – it can even be beneficial in certain situations – staying in a stress response long term can make you feel tired, sore, worried, anxious and overwhelmed.

In order to calm your mind and body back down, you need to counter the stress response with a 'relaxation response'. This will reduce your heart rate, so you feel less panicked. It also helps your muscles to loosen, which can ease pain and inflammation. As you relax, your brain will release

TELL A JOKE
Laughter can help you to relax, stimulating your circulation and easing your muscles.

Mindfulness for Men

endorphins, which make you feel better but also help to dull pain. There is some evidence to suggest that relaxing, and lowering stress hormones, can also help control your blood sugar level, strengthen your immune system and improve your sleep quality.

As you can see, spending time on specific relaxation techniques and activities is going to help improve your mindset and your wellbeing. The more you practise relaxation, the better you will get at it. So, if you don't feel the benefit right away, don't worry. Keep making time to relax and you will begin to feel better. Once you've nailed the techniques, you will be able to tap into those relaxing thoughts and feelings whenever you need to, giving you a toolkit to cope with stressful situations in the future.

HOW CAN WE RELAX MORE?

There are many different ways that you can bring relaxation into your life. It's quite personal seeing what works for you, so you may have to try a few things before you find the right activity or technique. Whatever you choose, give it time before deciding.

One way that you can relax is by introducing a form of meditation. We touched on this a little in the introduction to this book, by talking about a simple breath focus technique. That is a great place to start if you've

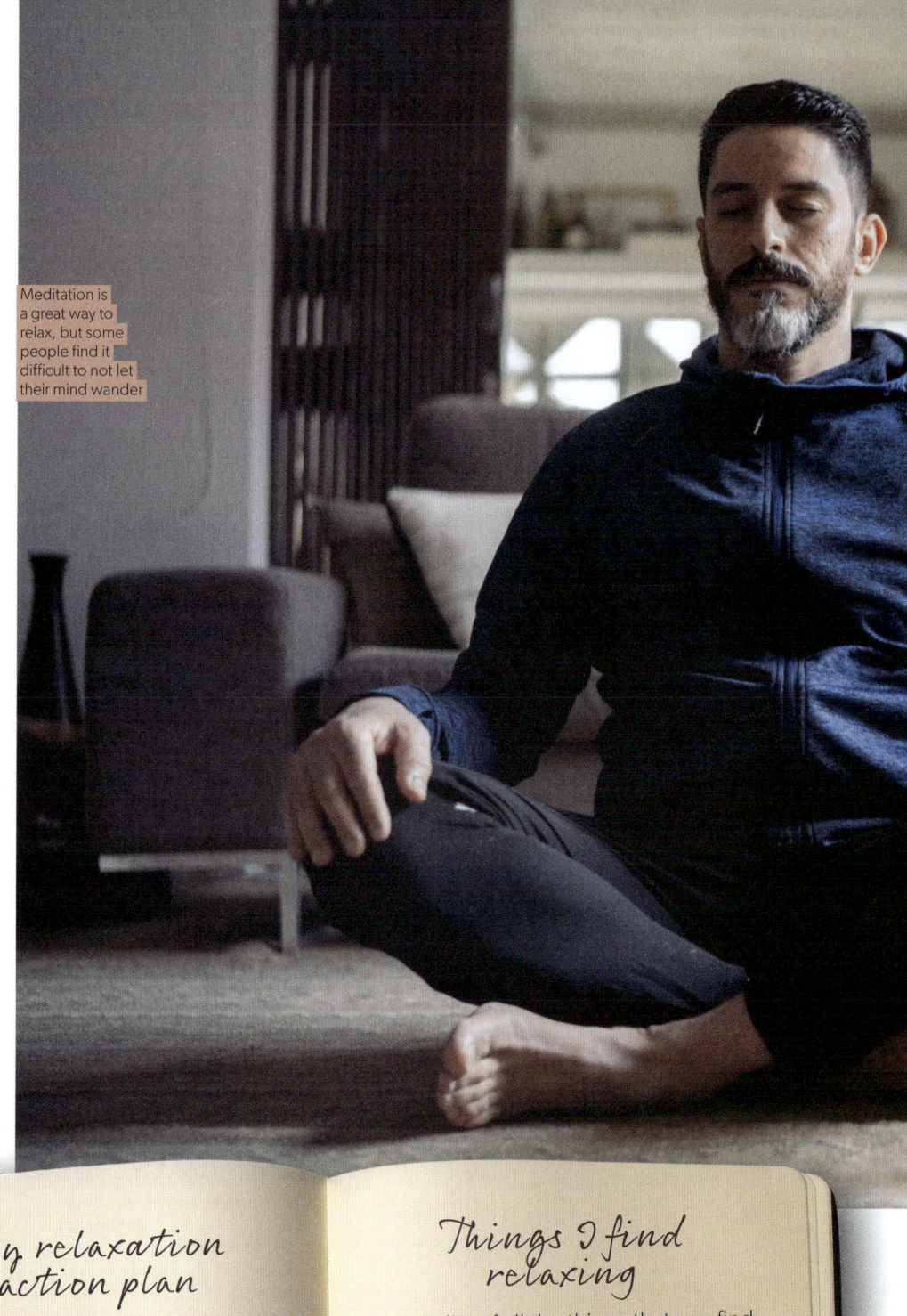

Meditation is a great way to relax, but some people find it difficult to not let their mind wander

My relaxation action plan

Use this space to write down what you will do to relax when you're feeling overwhelmed, stressed or worried. Refer back to it when you need to.

Things I find relaxing

Make a list of all the things that you find relaxing, then try to find time to do one or two of these each week.

Learn to relax

MONITOR YOUR HEART RATE

Your heart rate increases when you're stressed; when you relax, your heart rate will slow, helping your body recover.

to improve your mind-body connection by letting you tune into the way your body feels.

Guided meditations are available for free online. These often use imagery to help you focus and relax, such as imagining a relaxing scene in your mind. This can be a good exercise for those with a creative mindset and good imagination, making the scene as detailed as possible to help you ease into it. Some guided meditations will talk about a ball of light, a golden thread, or other forms of imagery to help you to focus.

You could also use meditation to focus on a specific mantra that means something to you – a prayer if you are religious or spiritual, or a gratitude for the day. As long as you are sitting still, and you're comfortable, focused and mindful, your body will begin to relax.

Of course, meditation isn't for everyone. You might prefer a more active form of regular relaxation, and many people turn to yoga or tai chi to achieve this. These practices incorporate a series of flowing moves that you work through while also controlling your breathing and your focus. For those who find their mind

The power of music

The right tunes can help to trigger a relaxation response, so set up a playlist!

When we listen to music, our bodies respond to the tempo of what we're listening to. If you listen to fast, upbeat music, it might make you feel energised and positive, which is great… just not when you're trying to relax. If you create a playlist of tunes you find soothing, this can help you switch off and relax whenever you need to. You want to look for music with a slower tempo, something that's around your natural resting heart rate, which can be anything from 40bpm (beats per minute) to 100bpm. Something around 60bpm is perfect for most people. If you use a service such as Spotify, there are playlists set up for most heart rates, so just search for '60 bpm' and see what your options are, or create your own playlist. Listening to calming, slower-tempo music can bring your heart rate down, making you feel relaxed and less stressed.

never done anything like this before. It's simple, doesn't require any investment, and just a couple of minutes a day can be enough to feel the benefits.

You can also try a body scan technique. Here, instead of solely focusing on your breath going in and out, you scan every part of your body with your mind. For each body part, tense the muscles and then let them relax completely, mentally directing your breath into that area. Work your way from your head to your toes, noticing any areas that are sore or stiff, and giving them your focus to relax. Again, this doesn't have to take very long, but it can help

Signs I need to relax

Think about what happens to your body and/or mind when you're stressed or worried. Do you feel tense, sore, angry? Write down the things you notice so you can become more mindful of when you need to make time to relax.

....

....

....

....

....

....

....

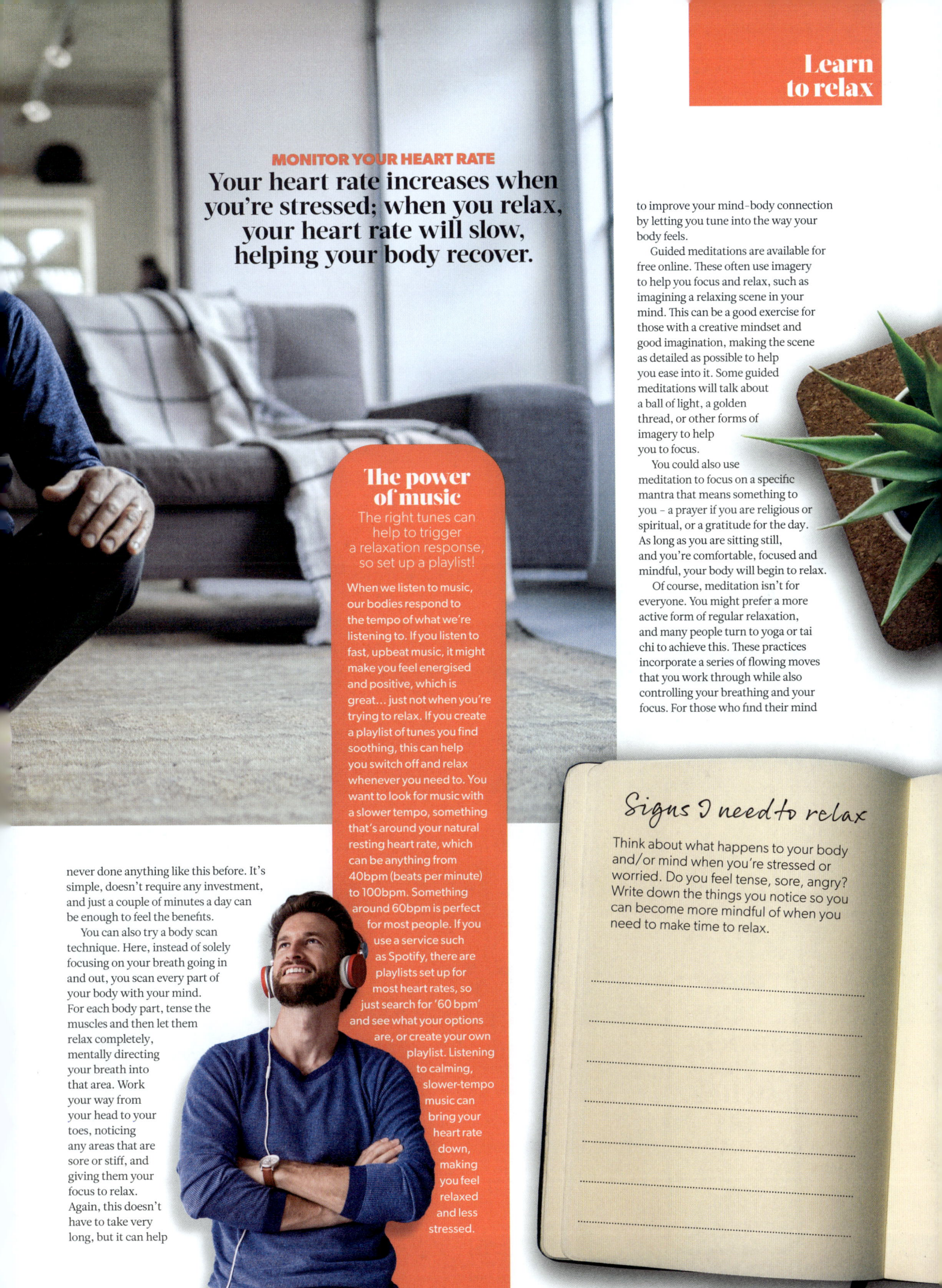

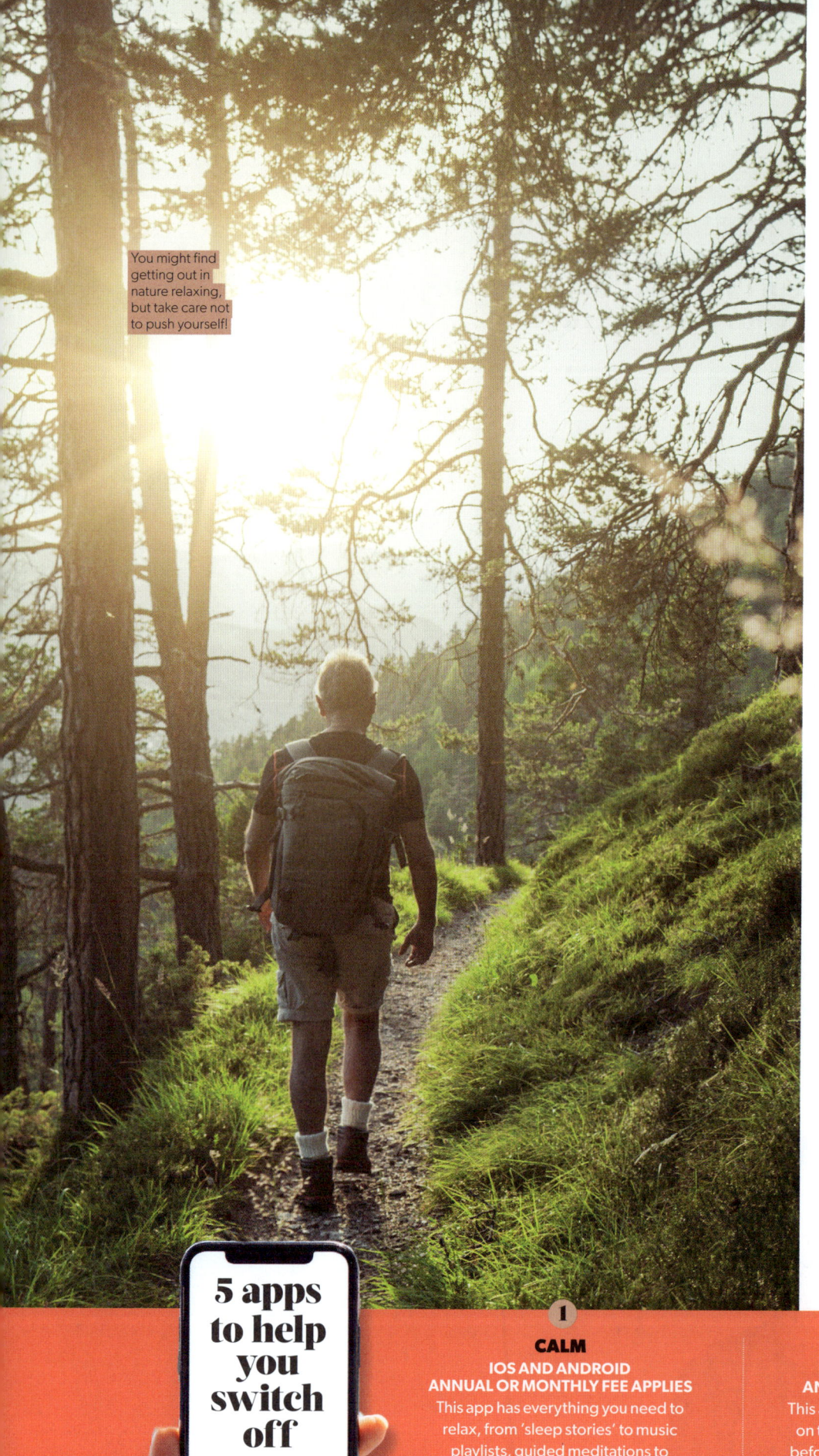

You might find getting out in nature relaxing, but take care not to push yourself!

wanders easily during meditation, doing yoga instead can help, as you are concentrating on the poses, leaving your mind free from intrusion. Some yoga styles are more intense than others, so if you're looking for a class, see if you can find one that is based on Hatha (a gentle style that focuses on flowing through the poses, or asanas) or Yin (a very slow-paced style where the asanas are held for longer). You can also find free yoga practices online, so you can do it in the comfort of your own home. Once you've learned the basics, you may choose to start or end your day with a few simple moves to relax.

Meditation and yoga are not the only ways to relax, but they are both very powerful and effective. However, you might prefer to relax in another way that suits you. For some, being outside in nature can trigger a relaxation response. This might be sitting in a local park, taking in your surroundings and breathing the air. You might prefer to walk gently and mindfully, so you're moving your body but not so much that you break a sweat – this isn't about physical exercise, it's about relaxation.

There are plenty of things that you can do at home too. You may like to curl up with a book and read. You might find unleashing your creativity to be relaxing, so why not do some colouring or doodling? Just let your pencil flow and try not to think too much about what you're doing – there's an activity to give this a go on the opposite page. You may find a warm bath relaxing, or simply sitting and watching a favourite film.

The main thing to take away from this is that you need to find time to fit relaxation into your life. A few minutes per day is much better than a longer session once a fortnight. Think about where you can do something relaxing in your current schedule, and try to stick to it. Hopefully, within a couple of weeks, you'll really start to feel the benefits.

5 apps to help you switch off

Make your tech work for you with these handy smartphone apps

1
CALM
IOS AND ANDROID
ANNUAL OR MONTHLY FEE APPLIES
This app has everything you need to relax, from 'sleep stories' to music playlists, guided meditations to gratitude check-ins. It has a Daily Calm feature, which is different every day, to help you build a routine around relaxation, plus there are more than 100 guided meditations.

2
HEADSPACE
IOS AND ANDROID
ANNUAL OR MONTHLY FEE APPLIES
This app is probably one of the best known on the market right now. It has a free trial before you start a subscription, so you can see what it offers. It has daily meditations, including three-minute mini meditations, as well as sleep sounds, relaxing meditations, anxiety- and stress-relief meditations, and breathwork practices.

Learn to relax

Do a doodle

Doodling can help you to relax, so use this space to freely draw whatever comes to mind. Don't overthink it; just let your pencil flow and see what happens

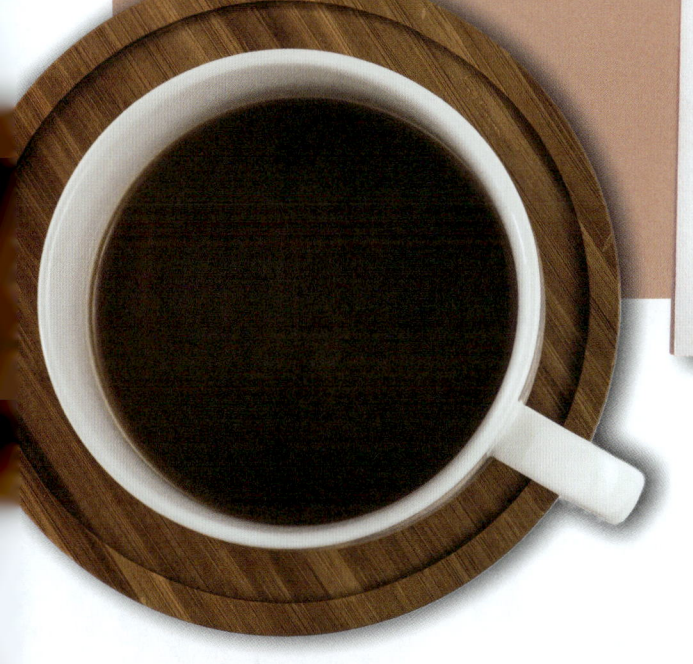

VISUALISE YOUR CALM

Close your eyes and think about a place where you feel most calm. Your happy place. Think of the details and use all your senses.

3
SIMPLE HABIT
IOS AND ANDROID
ANNUAL OR MONTHLY FEE APPLIES

For those who are really busy, this app helps you to relax in just five minutes, to reduce stress and improve sleep quality. It tracks your progress and reminds you to take the time to relax, whether it's when you wake up, during a commute in the car or before sleep. There are themed meditations for everything you might be experiencing in your life at any given time.

4
COLORFY
IOS AND ANDROID
FREE, WITH IN-APP PURCHASES

If you're looking for something completely different and creative, then this could be for you. It's a digital colouring book for adults, with lots of creation options and brush types. It works well on a phone, but you might prefer the larger screen of a tablet for this. You can also use it offline, so it's accessible all the time.

5
NATURESPACE
IOS AND ANDROID
FREE, WITH IN-APP PURCHASES

This simple app has high-quality sounds to help you create a relaxing environment. The sounds have been recorded in the real world and are designed for specific uses, such as sleep, working, stress relief and meditation. It can help you to block out any distracting noises. You get six free tracks to start off with, then you purchase any additional tracks you want.

Mindfulness for Men

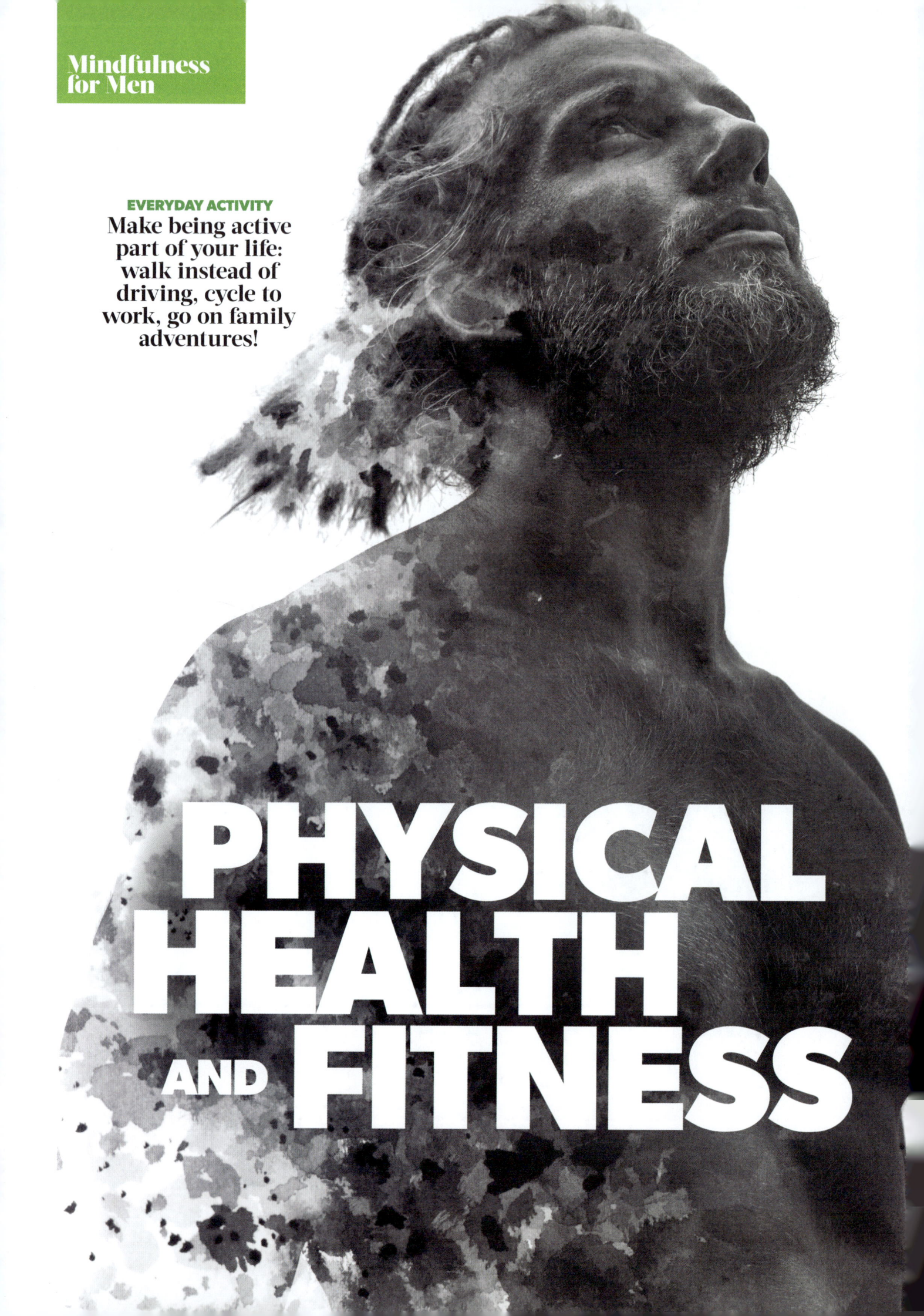

EVERYDAY ACTIVITY
Make being active part of your life: walk instead of driving, cycle to work, go on family adventures!

PHYSICAL HEALTH AND FITNESS

Being mindful around fitness can help you to improve your relationship with exercise and boost your wellbeing

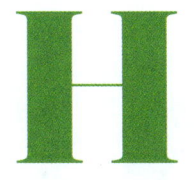

My current physical health

Use this space to write down how you feel about your physical health right now. Do you have any conditions or ailments to consider? Do you feel strong in some areas? Do you perceive any weaknesses?

....
....
....
....
....
....

How do you feel physically right now? Would you describe yourself as being in good health? Do you feel fit and strong? Or are you struggling with health conditions, injuries or illness?

There are no right or wrong answers here. What we're asking is for you to be truly honest about your physical health and fitness as it stands in this moment. Try this mindful activity: scan your body from head to toe and consider each body part, thinking about how different areas feel and perform. Note down where you feel strong, whether that's powerful legs from exercise, or good balance, or great stamina. Also note down areas where you feel less strong, which could include medical conditions that impact your physical health (asthma, IBS, tendonitis and so on), as well as muscles you don't feel you use very often or low cardio fitness levels. There's space on these pages for you to write down your thoughts.

When everything is going well, it's easy to take health for granted. There's often a trigger that causes us to ask questions about our current health, and whether we can make any changes. For those who are active, it can be an injury that forces us to stop and rest, then have to consider how we build back up again. Or it might be the diagnosis of a specific medical condition that gives us the perspective we need to want to improve our health and fitness. Reading this now, you might have reached one of these trigger points and be ready to make changes to your physical health and fitness, or you might have never really considered auditing your body in this way before.

Once you've done an initial scan and identified where you feel your current health and fitness is at, you can start to make a plan of action – we've included space on pages 78-79 for you to note down your future goals. It can be tempting to throw yourself into the gym or sign up for a big event, but as well as being mindful about your physical health and fitness, you can also be more mindful about the exercise you choose to engage in. Crafting the perfect fitness regime for you will reap much greater benefits than simply following a 'one-size-fits-all' training programme.

BENEFITS OF BEING MORE MINDFUL ABOUT PHYSICAL HEALTH

There are lots of positives to being mindful around your physical health and fitness. For a start, by being mindful of your body, you can stop yourself from overdoing it. If you try to tackle a problem head-on, and go from doing nothing to doing everything, you're asking for an injury. Being mindful means being aware of your body. Learn when you need to take a rest day and when you feel like you can go hard. By being mindful, you will learn the best ways to recover for you – this might be anything from knowing you can't run on back-to-back days or that you need to stretch every day, to becoming aware of how much sleep you need each night to maintain your physical health and do the exercise you want to do.

Another benefit of being mindful in this area is being able to determine what you enjoy and what you don't. There are so many options out there for maintaining fitness and they won't all suit you. It's easy to get drawn into the mindset that you have to go to the gym to get strong, or that you have to run to boost your cardio health, but neither of these are true.

The basic guidelines (as suggested by both the NHS in the UK and the US Department of Health and Human Services), says that adults should aim for around 150 minutes per week of moderate intensity activity, or 75 minutes of vigorous activity, as well as strengthening activities that work all the major muscle groups on at least two days a week. What the guidance doesn't say is how you have to achieve that. For your cardio activity, you could run, walk fast, climb mountains, cycle,

Mindful movement

Slow down to maximise the benefits of an exercise regime

If your idea of exercise is to get as much done in as short a time as possible, then you might not be getting all the benefits that you could be. Try making sure that some of your sessions are slower, and that you perform concentrated movements that you have to focus on. This can be applied to any form of exercise. If you like lifting in the gym, do some workouts where you focus on one technique and drill down into the skills you need. Perform the move, analyse how you did it and make tweaks. If you like to run, make at least one session much slower than your normal pace and use the time to focus on your running form, thinking about your foot placement and your centre of gravity. If you find it hard to slow down, then consider adding in a yoga class or tai chi to your routine, where you need to tune in to your body and concentrate on getting the movements correct.

77

Mindfulness for Men

Right: The gym is an obvious place to go to improve your health, but rather than mindlessly run through exercises, take time to focus on the movements you make and how your body and muscles feel

Acknowledge your limitations

While physical health and fitness are connected, there are issues that can impact your health and wellbeing outside of exercise

Being mindful about your physical health means acknowledging any ailments or medical conditions that have an impact on your body. If you have a specific condition that limits you in some way, it can be hard to feel as if you have much power over your physical health and wellness. However, mindfulness can help you to become more accepting of any limitations, and also help you to explore positive solutions and adaptations to move in different ways.

Some ailments might only be temporary, such as injuries, which are often frustrating but usually heal with time. If this is the case, spend some time thinking about your injury and what you need to do to help your body heal. It might be that you can't exercise right now, but you could spend some extra time on meditation, hobbies or self-care to help bolster your physical health in other ways.

Try to focus on what you can do, and not what you can't. If you're a runner who can't currently run, maybe this is your chance to work on your flexibility and strength, for example.

Other medical conditions can be more limiting, but they still form part of our physical health. For those living with chronic illness, it can be overwhelming, frustrating and isolating. By practising mindfulness, we can learn to recognise these feelings and validate them. We can then practise accepting these feelings and finding different ways to respond to them. Having a medical condition doesn't mean that better physical health is out of reach; we might just have to set different parameters around what we want to achieve. The goal is to consider the best physical health that you, personally, can achieve and the steps you need to take to get there.

---

play golf, go to a gym class, try boxing, play tennis, go swimming... For your strength work, you might like to try weightlifting, bodyweight circuits, yoga or Pilates. You can also work all your muscles through things like digging in the garden or doing DIY tasks – sports aren't the only way to get fit! The point is that you can opt to do whatever exercise you like, and if you enjoy it, then you're more likely to do it.

This is great if you have a bad relationship with exercise – many of us are impacted by past experiences and put off from trying new things. By implanting a more mindful attitude towards exercise, you can be true to what you actually want to do while still reaping the rewards. Bear that in mind during your fitness journey; be honest with yourself about whether you are really enjoying something or you're only doing it because your feel you 'have' to. There is always another option out there that might help you reach your goals.

There are advantages that come from an enhanced awareness of your current fitness. If you have identified areas in which you need to improve, you can start to apply changes. So, if you know that you find going for a walk leaves you a little breathless, your goal might be to gently increase your cardio fitness by committing to taking more walks for longer periods of time, and logging your improvements over time. We know that exercise has huge benefits, and holding these benefits in your mind can help keep you motivated. Being physically fit can reduce your risk of some major

SIT LESS
Reduce the time you spend sitting, and break up inactive periods with movement in order to kickstart your physical health goals.

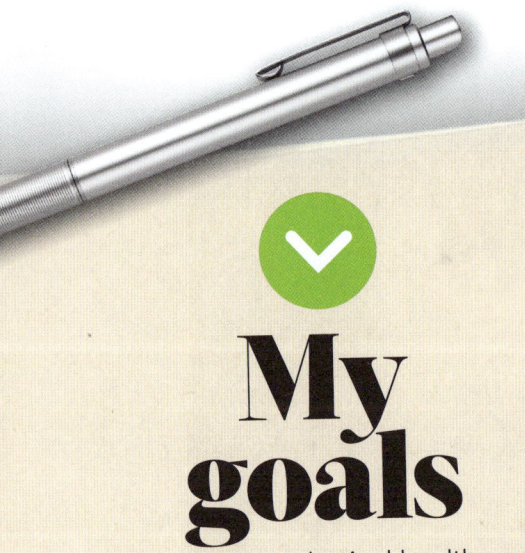

My goals

Let's set some physical health goals! This can be anything you want to achieve, such as a weight goal, a specific fitness goal (e.g. run a 5K), a lifestyle goal (e.g. being able to play football with the kids for an hour) or anything else you think of.

My goal

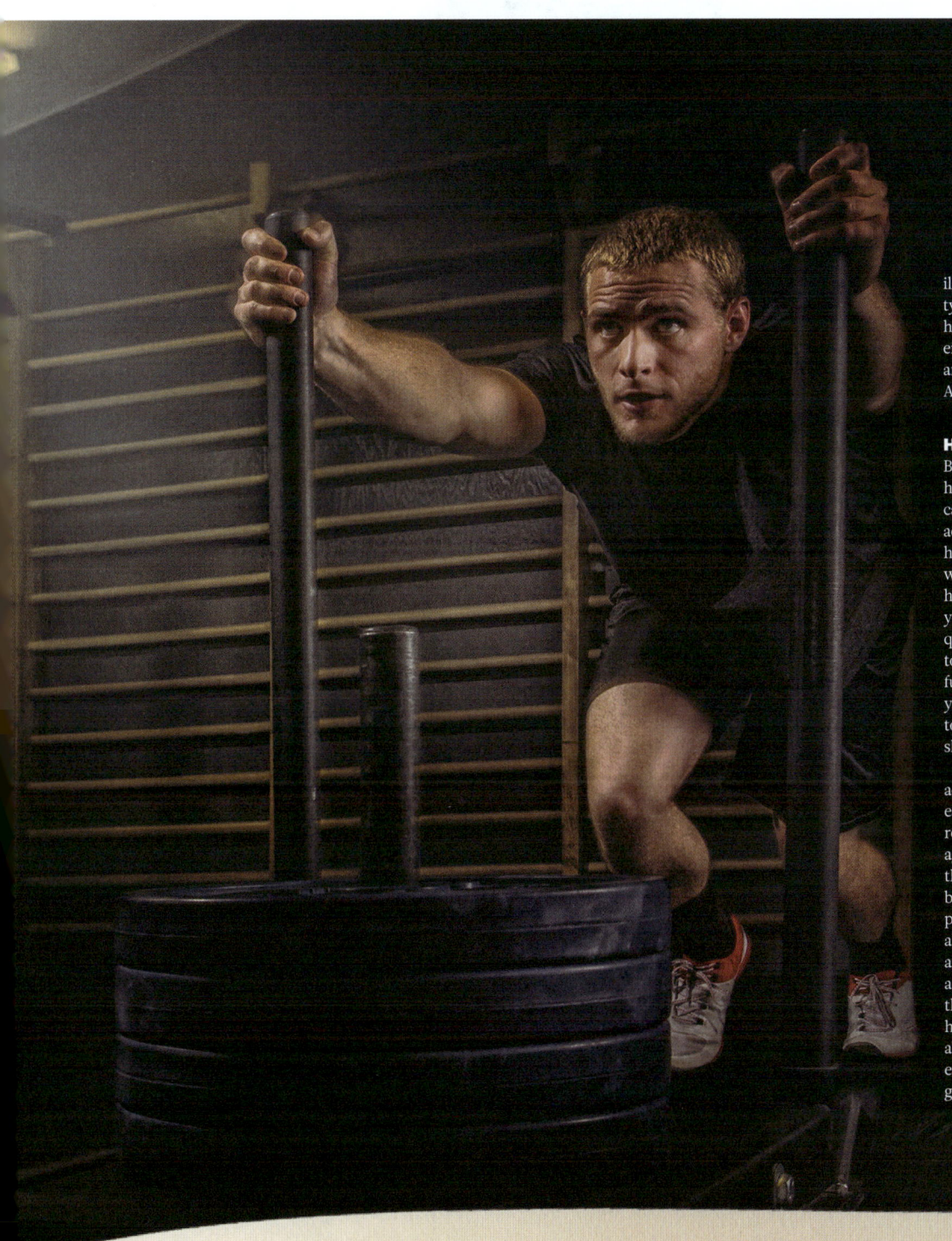

Physical health and fitness

illnesses, such as heart disease, stroke, type 2 diabetes and cancer. It can also help you to sleep better, increase your energy, boost your mood, relieve stress, and reduce your risk of dementia and Alzheimer's disease.

HOW TO GET STARTED
Being mindful around your physical health and fitness is something everyone can do, no matter what your current activity level. Hopefully by this point, you have identified some areas you feel you would like to work on and maybe even have an idea of what kind of activities you might like to do. If you're already quite active and fit, then you may want to think about how you'd like to progress further, any changes you want to make to your routine, or new activities you'd like to incorporate, or create a back-up plan should you get ill or injured in the future.

The next step is to engage in those activities in a mindful manner. It's very easy to just turn up at a gym, follow a routine through mindlessly, and go home again, ticking off another workout. Sure, that will help you increase your fitness, but you can get more out of it. Try to stay present in all of your sessions – think about what you are doing and why you are doing it. Focus on the muscle you are working at that moment, and notice the resistance – could you push a little harder, or do you need to back off? Think about your 'why' to help you through each workout. After you've finished, it's good to reflect on the session and think

Why I'd like to achieve this goal

Target completion date

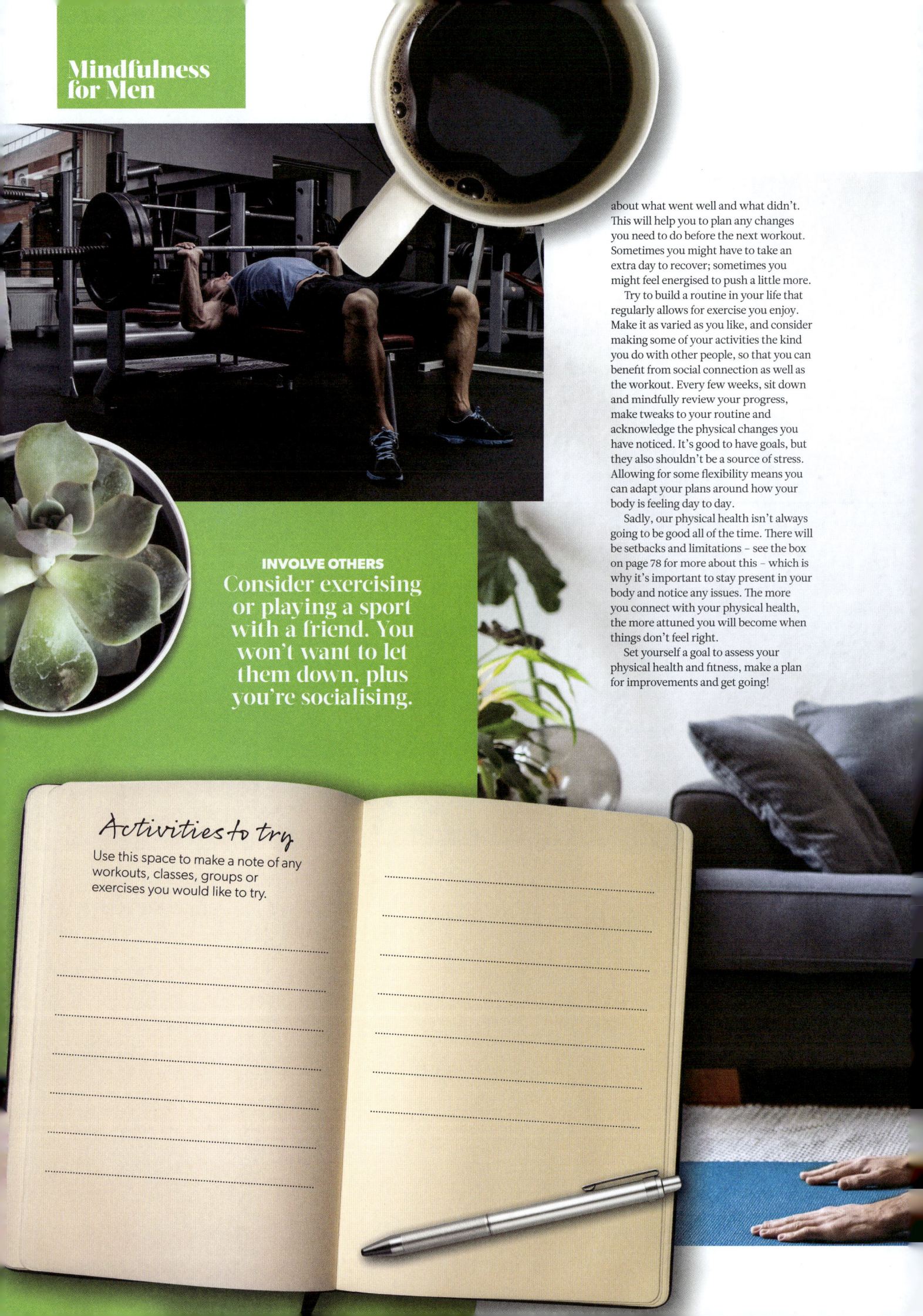

Mindfulness for Men

about what went well and what didn't. This will help you to plan any changes you need to do before the next workout. Sometimes you might have to take an extra day to recover; sometimes you might feel energised to push a little more.

Try to build a routine in your life that regularly allows for exercise you enjoy. Make it as varied as you like, and consider making some of your activities the kind you do with other people, so that you can benefit from social connection as well as the workout. Every few weeks, sit down and mindfully review your progress, make tweaks to your routine and acknowledge the physical changes you have noticed. It's good to have goals, but they also shouldn't be a source of stress. Allowing for some flexibility means you can adapt your plans around how your body is feeling day to day.

Sadly, our physical health isn't always going to be good all of the time. There will be setbacks and limitations – see the box on page 78 for more about this – which is why it's important to stay present in your body and notice any issues. The more you connect with your physical health, the more attuned you will become when things don't feel right.

Set yourself a goal to assess your physical health and fitness, make a plan for improvements and get going!

INVOLVE OTHERS
Consider exercising or playing a sport with a friend. You won't want to let them down, plus you're socialising.

Activities to try
Use this space to make a note of any workouts, classes, groups or exercises you would like to try.

Physical health and fitness

My weekly fitness routine

Plan out a weekly fitness routine that you would like to follow to improve your physical health. Make sure you vary your workouts, and include some mindful movement (such as yoga or stretching) and some rest days.

Day	Planned activity
Monday	
Tuesday	
Wednesday	
Thursday	
Friday	
Saturday	
Sunday	

Don't forget to include mindful activities such as yoga into your exercise routine

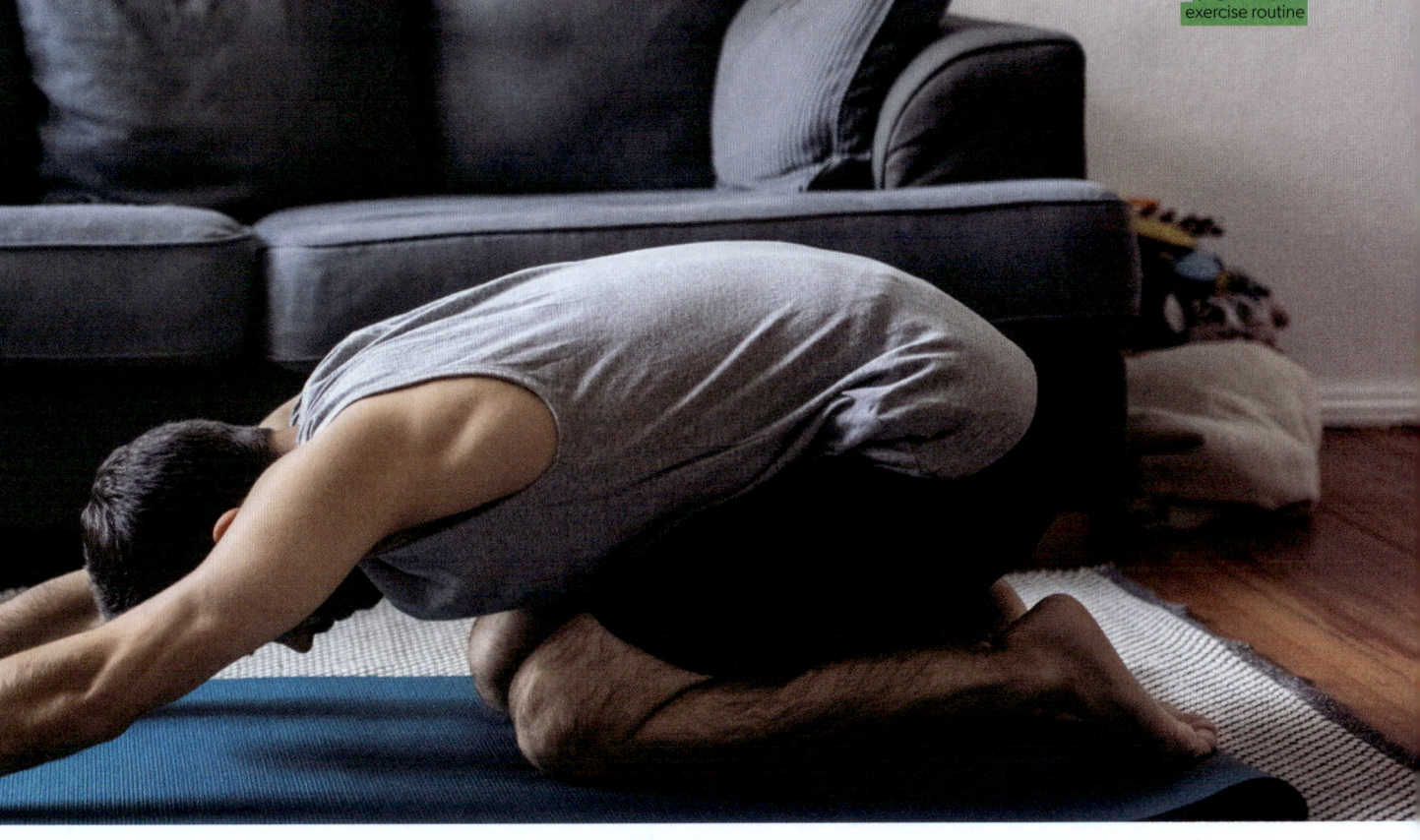

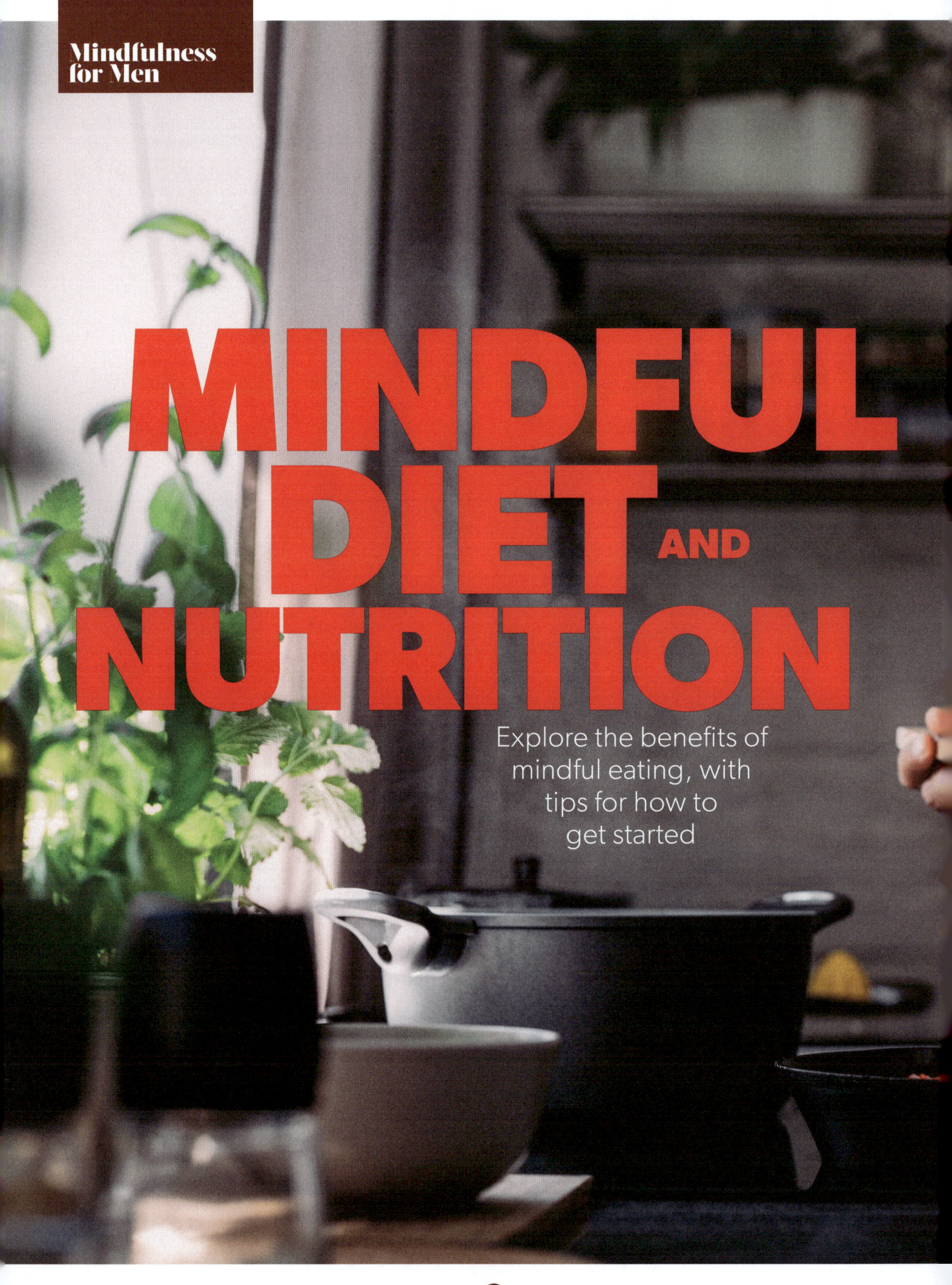

Mindfulness for Men

MINDFUL DIET AND NUTRITION

Explore the benefits of mindful eating, with tips for how to get started

Mindful diet and nutrition

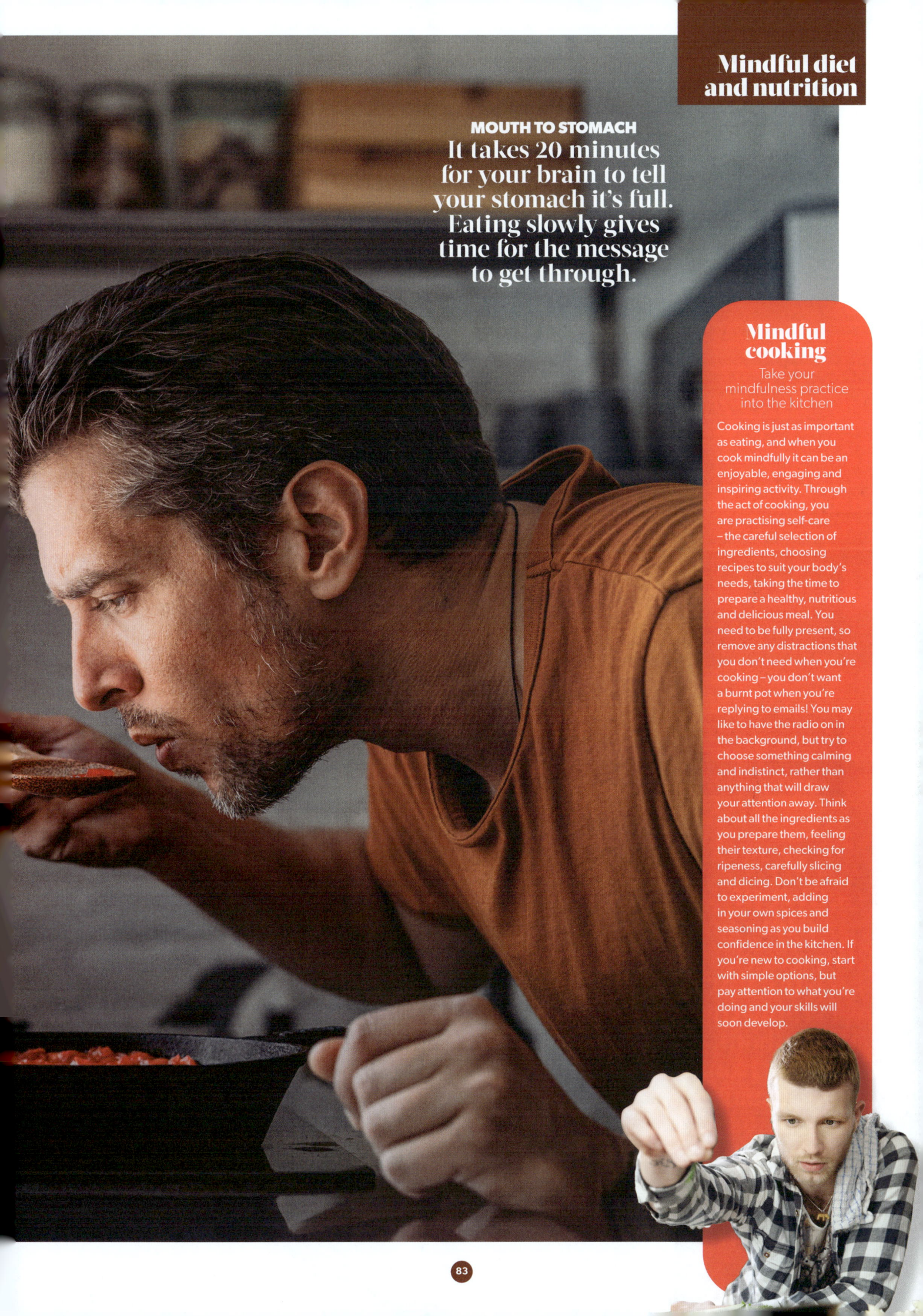

MOUTH TO STOMACH
It takes 20 minutes for your brain to tell your stomach it's full. Eating slowly gives time for the message to get through.

Mindful cooking
Take your mindfulness practice into the kitchen

Cooking is just as important as eating, and when you cook mindfully it can be an enjoyable, engaging and inspiring activity. Through the act of cooking, you are practising self-care – the careful selection of ingredients, choosing recipes to suit your body's needs, taking the time to prepare a healthy, nutritious and delicious meal. You need to be fully present, so remove any distractions that you don't need when you're cooking – you don't want a burnt pot when you're replying to emails! You may like to have the radio on in the background, but try to choose something calming and indistinct, rather than anything that will draw your attention away. Think about all the ingredients as you prepare them, feeling their texture, checking for ripeness, carefully slicing and dicing. Don't be afraid to experiment, adding in your own spices and seasoning as you build confidence in the kitchen. If you're new to cooking, start with simple options, but pay attention to what you're doing and your skills will soon develop.

Mindfulness for Men

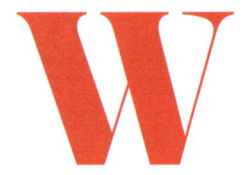

What you eat and how you eat it can have a great impact on your mental health and wellbeing. It's not about any one specific diet, however. It's about being mindful around food and acknowledging what you're choosing to put into your body. In this feature, we'll be exploring how to pay attention to what you eat and drink, and how this mindfulness around diet can have wide-ranging benefits.

In the modern, busy world that we live in, food can become a rushed experience. We might grab breakfast as we fly out the door or while we're preparing food for family members; lunch might be at our desks or skipped entirely; we might reach for a sugary snack mid-afternoon for an energy boost; and dinner can be grabbed in a hurry or eaten in front of the TV. There are also other reasons why someone might eat, besides being hungry. It could be that you eat for comfort or out of boredom, or you might have associated certain foods with non-mealtime activities, such as eating popcorn at the cinema. Of course, you might not be guilty of all or any of these, but we all have moments where we eat mindlessly,

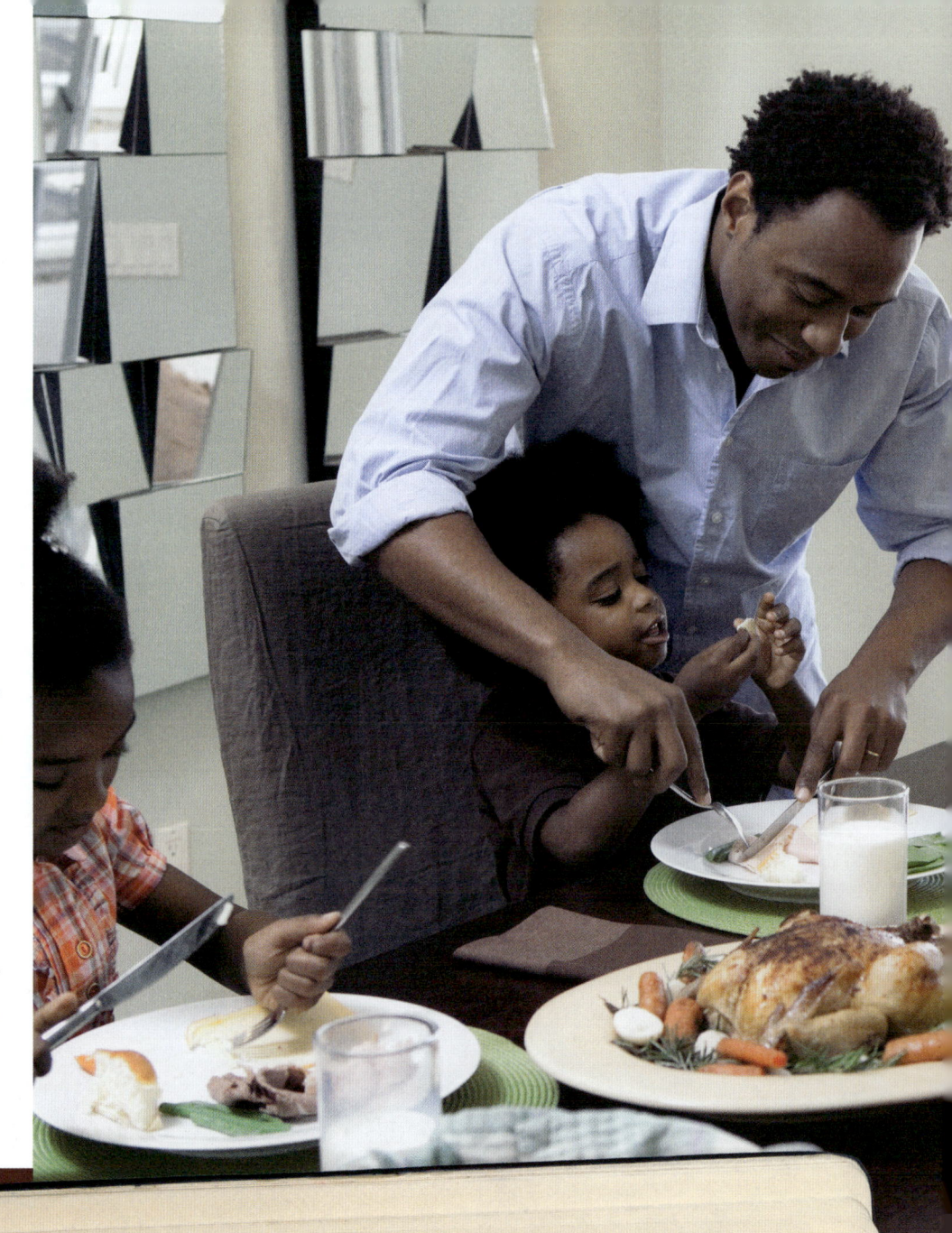

> My current diet

For a week, keep track of everything you eat without deviating from your usual eating pattern, so you can analyse your current diet.

	Breakfast	Lunch	Dinner	Snacks
Monday				
Tuesday				
Wednesday				
Thursday				
Friday				
Saturday				
Sunday				

Recipes to try

Use this space to write down a recipe you would like to try to cook in the future, then commit to buying the ingredients and cooking it mindfully this month.

....

....

....

....

....

....

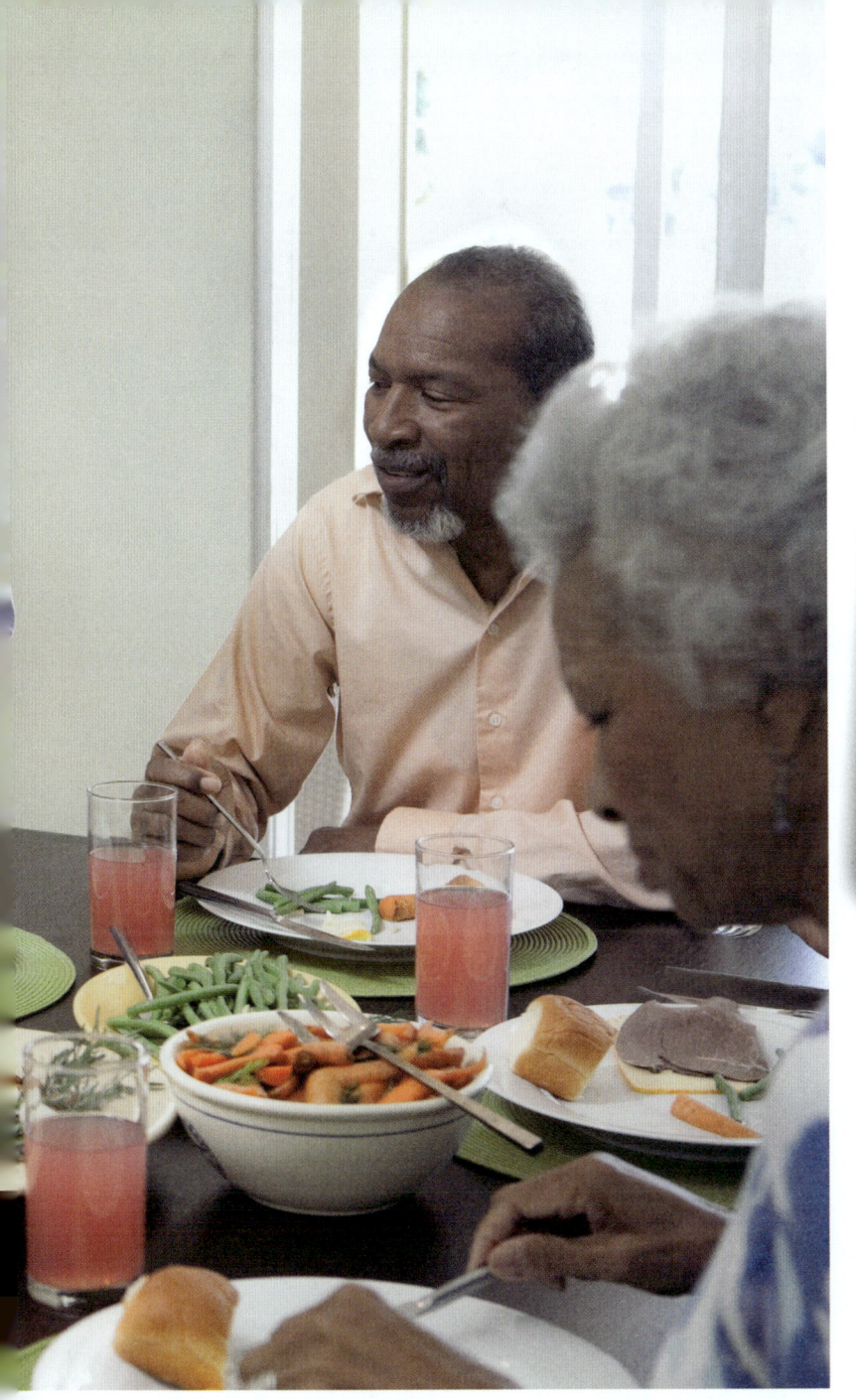

distracted or with no thought given to the food we're consuming.

Mindful eating isn't about giving anything up; it isn't about eating only 'healthy' foods or never choosing the easy option. You can still order a takeaway; you're just doing so mindfully and with full awareness. It's not a restrictive diet and there are no limitations, but by becoming more aware of what you are eating and drinking, you may find that you naturally gravitate towards good choices. Like all aspects of mindfulness, mindful eating is about being 'in the moment' when it comes to food and drink. It's about understanding what food you choose to eat, how it makes you feel, what it tastes like and why you enjoy it.

HOW TO BE MORE MINDFUL ABOUT DIET AND NUTRITION

When you first start thinking about eating in a more mindful manner, you may find it useful to keep some kind of food diary. This helps you to introduce some accountability and awareness of how you behave around food. You don't have to change anything in your diet for now. Simply take a moment before you eat or drink to note down what you're consuming; if you prefer, you could just take a picture. This forces you to look at what you're eating and really acknowledge it. Once you've had your meal or snack, it's also useful to write down a couple of bullet points about how it made you feel. Do you feel full? Satisfied? Bloated? Uncomfortable? Happy? Did you enjoy the food? Also think about why you were eating the food, especially if it's not a mealtime. Were you feeling stressed and wanted something to help calm you, or were you bored and needed something to do?

Try this for a week without changing anything – this gives you a chance to be honest and analyse your current diet and nutrition. Then, when you've spent a little time on this exercise, review your food diary and analyse how it makes you feel. You might find specific patterns around eating; for example, if you eat late at night, you sleep less well. Only when you become truly mindful around your diet, will you be able to see these kinds of triggers and the impact that your nutritional choices are having on other areas of your life.

Once you've looked at your current diet and nutrition, you can then start to use the principles of mindfulness to make the changes you need to. But do be aware that you can't change everything immediately, and don't be too hard on yourself. If you have a busy family life or long working hours, you're not going to have time to always prepare meals from scratch, sit down at a table and eat at a set time. However, you can still bring aspects of mindful eating into your diet, even when you're rushed off your feet and darting about everywhere.

Being more mindful about your diet and nutrition means looking at your relationship with food, and for some people this can be an uncomfortable experience. If you use food to help in times of stress or emotional distress, you need to be sure that you have another way of coping in these situations, whether that's going for a walk, taking time to read a book, watching a TV show, or having a warm shower. If you eat

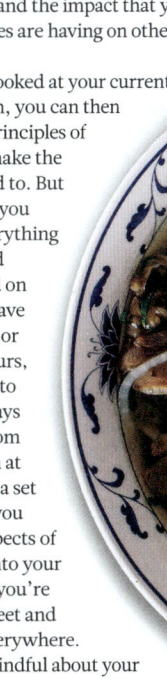

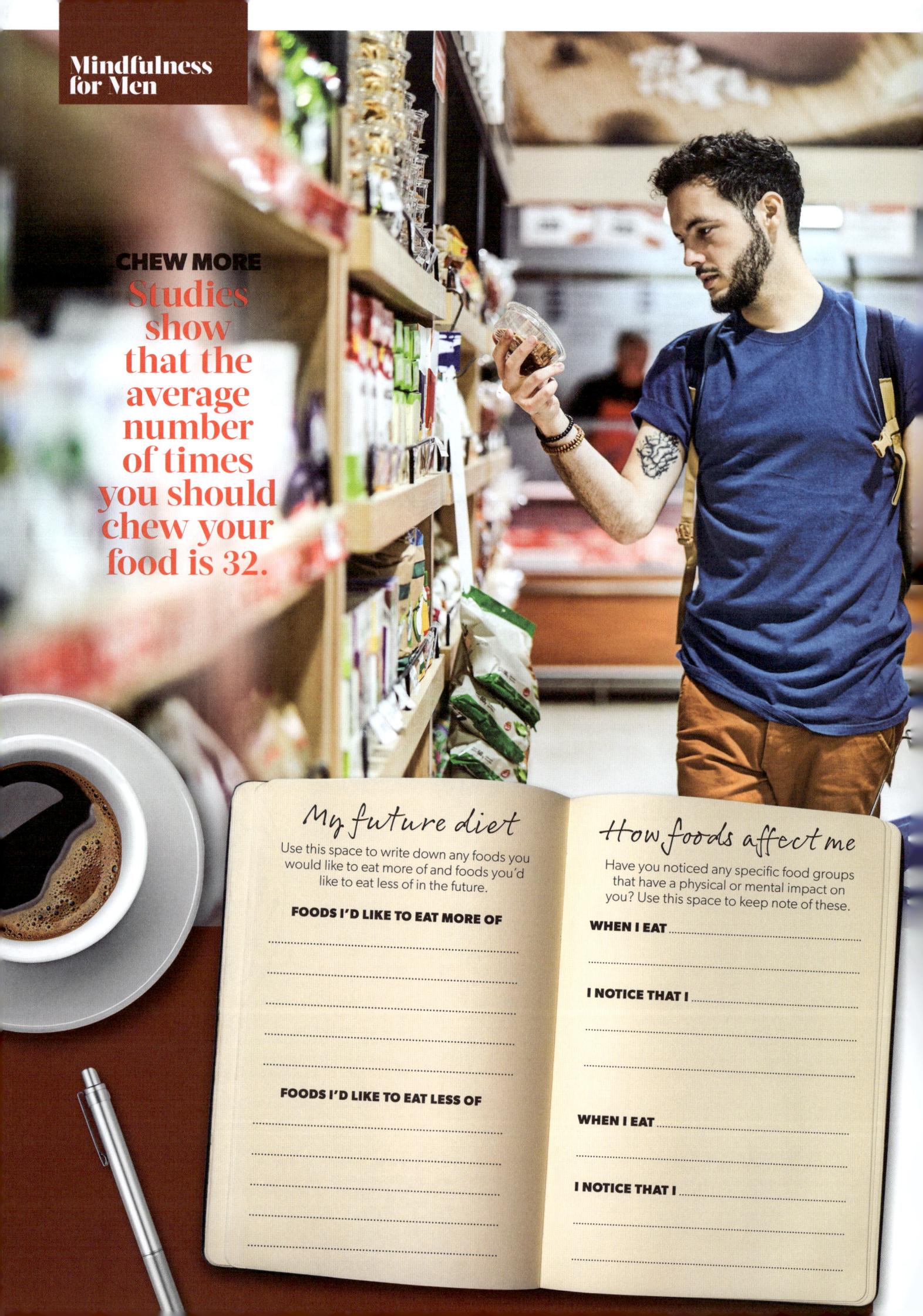

Mindfulness for Men

CHEW MORE
Studies show that the average number of times you should chew your food is 32.

My future diet
Use this space to write down any foods you would like to eat more of and foods you'd like to eat less of in the future.

FOODS I'D LIKE TO EAT MORE OF
....
....
....
....

FOODS I'D LIKE TO EAT LESS OF
....
....
....
....

How foods affect me
Have you noticed any specific food groups that have a physical or mental impact on you? Use this space to keep note of these.

WHEN I EAT ....
....

I NOTICE THAT I ....
....
....
....

WHEN I EAT ....
....

I NOTICE THAT I ....
....
....

Food cravings and how to beat them

Banish food cravings once and for all by applying mindful principles

Food cravings can be the downfall of good intentions for many of us. You may experience a very intense desire for a certain food, so much so that it takes over your thoughts and you won't be satisfied until you consume it. For others, it might be an intruding thought that's more easily pushed aside. However, we all only have so much willpower, and the more cravings you have, the more likely it is that you will eventually give in to them.

When a craving comes, the first thing to do is acknowledge it. For example, you may feel a powerful craving for sugar when you're tired. Notice that craving and bring your awareness to it. Recognise that you're only craving that food because you are tired, then explore what other options you have for dealing with the problem. A large glass of cold water can have the effect of waking you up. A walk around the block in the fresh air can also help you to feel more alert, and sometimes you may need to take a moment to relax or even have a short nap. If you find that the craving is still there, you might want to try eating something different instead. So, rather than reaching for a biscuit to alleviate your craving, try a piece of fruit and focus on the sweetness of it.

You might also find that with other lifestyle changes, you have fewer cravings. Make sure you're getting plenty of sleep, eating enough protein, not getting too hungry between meals and exercising regularly.

when you're bored rather than when you're hungry, have some activities to hand to replace food.

The key thing is to really think about what you're choosing to eat and drink. Consider how a food tastes and how it makes you feel. Appreciate the food you have and take the time to slow down and enjoy it.

HOW TO PRACTISE MINDFUL EATING

It's best to start small and build up, so maybe identify one meal a day where you have the time and space to be mindful about what you eat. Prepare your meal with care, thinking about the food you're choosing to eat and why you're choosing to eat it. Make it look attractive on your plate to trigger your sense of sight and smell. Think about adding plenty of colour and textures to make the food interesting. Consider how hungry you are feeling when plating up – it's often better to start with less and go back for more if you're still hungry.

Next, try to eat at a table without any distractions. This helps you to focus on eating and only eating. Take a moment before you begin to acknowledge your meal, and to enjoy the aroma of your food. This can help to build into the anticipation and enjoyment of the meal. When you start eating, make sure you take a bite and chew it properly so that you can think about its texture, taste and flavour. Continue eating, but try to be mindful of how full you are feeling and stop when you feel your body has had enough. You don't have to eat beyond comfort – over time, you will be better in tune with your body and will be able to anticipate how much to plate up, but in the early days, don't be afraid to leave food when you're finished.

Eating mindfully is something that can be done with others. If you're eating a family meal at home, try to involve everyone in picking recipes and helping prepare it, or serving it 'family style' in the middle of the table for everyone to help themselves. Talk about the food and how it tastes, and use the time to connect as well as to eat. In a restaurant, take the time to appreciate the skill that has gone into making your meal, especially if it's something you wouldn't typically prepare at home.

Mindful eating incorporates the entire process of food, from source to plate. When shopping for ingredients, if you can go in person, look at the quality and texture of fresh fruits and vegetables, read packaging to understand what you're buying, and be mindful about everything you put in your basket. The cooking process can be incredibly mindful, and many find it relaxing and enjoyable.

THE BENEFITS OF MINDFUL EATING

Eating more mindfully can have huge benefits. When you dial into how food makes you feel, you may find yourself drawn to foods that are better for your body. We all know that we need to eat plenty of fruit and veg, sources of protein, complex carbohydrates and small amounts of healthy fats. We also know that we should limit processed foods, sugar and saturated fat. You may find that you gravitate towards a healthier diet just by being aware of what you are putting on your plate. By focusing on what's on your plate for each meal, you will notice patterns where you lack certain food groups or types, so you can mindfully introduce them into your diet.

Slowing down when eating has been shown to aid with digestion, which can help with inflammatory conditions like IBS, as well as bloating after meals. Learning about your own hunger cues can mean that you eat less in each sitting, giving your body just what it needs, which is beneficial to maintaining a healthy weight. It can help you with changing your relationship with food, understanding how you need it to fuel your body, and improve your wellbeing. You may also find that you enjoy your food more, as you really take the time to taste and smell, learning what you like. The simple act of stopping for a meal can encourage you to take regular breaks in a busy schedule, which can help to manage stress and anxiety. It can also build and foster relationships if you eat with others.

Mindful eating isn't a fad diet or something that you do for a short period of time; it's a lifelong change to the way you approach your diet and nutrition.

Mindfulness for Men

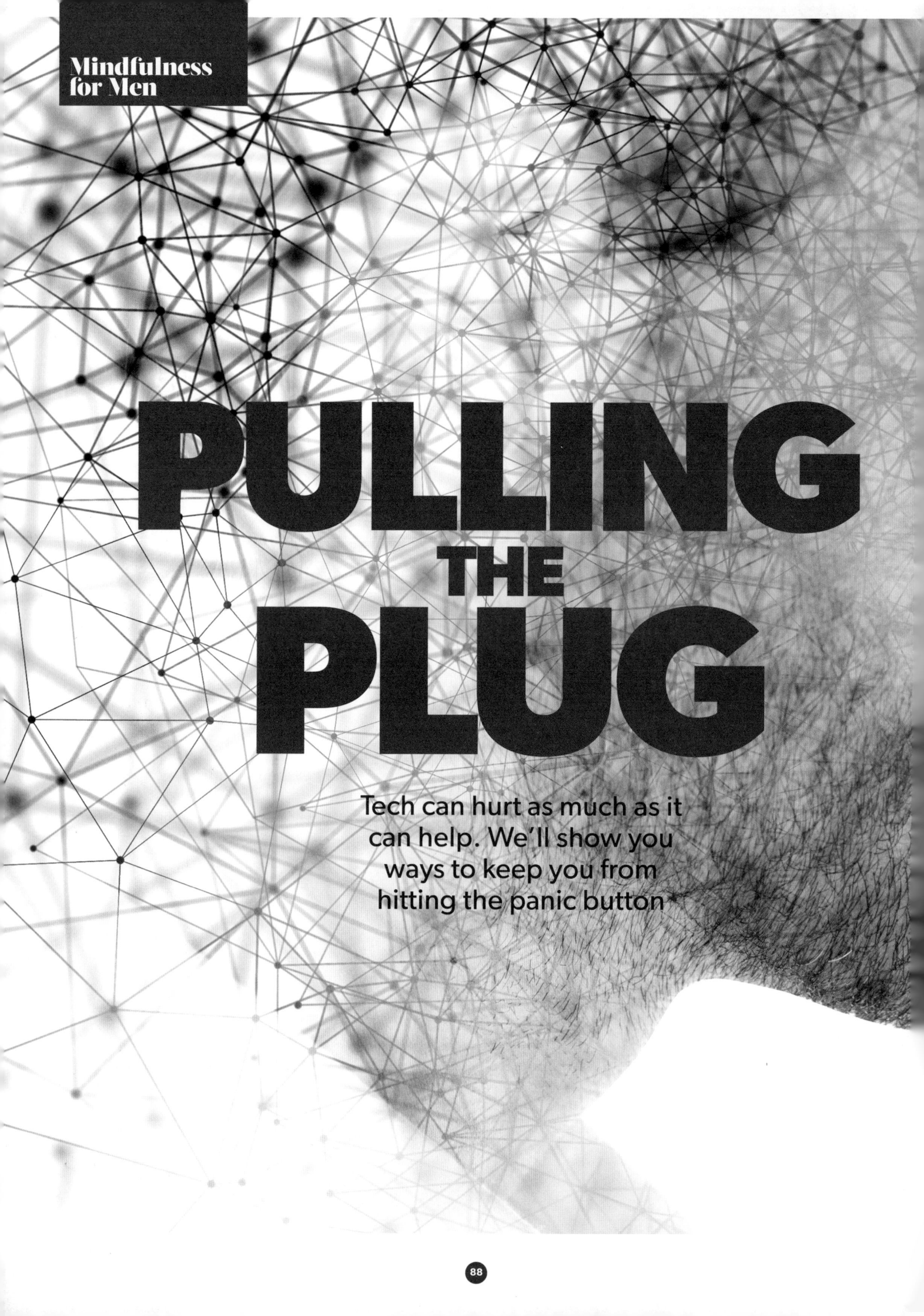

PULLING THE PLUG

Tech can hurt as much as it can help. We'll show you ways to keep you from hitting the panic button

Pulling the plug

It's impossible to picture modern life without the comfort of computers, tablets, smartphones, streaming-capable TVs and game consoles. Today, technology permeates our entire day: we reach for our devices as soon as we wake up and only set them down when it's time to go to sleep.

As helpful as it can be in streamlining our lives and making us feel more connected than any other generation before us, technology is like a double-edged sword that can harm as much as it can help, if used recklessly.

Now, we can imagine some of you read that last sentence and rolled your eyes, but there's no denying that social media and gaming addictions are very much real and should be handled seriously. Additionally, the pressure of omnipresent work, online FOMO and social media validation can negatively affect your self-esteem and feed anxiety.

Because our devices are ever-present, it's tough to shut off – especially when you consider certain apps are specifically designed to hold your attention. Let's face it, many of us have spent needlessly late nights aimlessly scrolling through Twitter, TikTok or Tinder, not really knowing what we're looking for.

That's not to say you should quit using your devices and chuck them in the bin. Rather, if you become more aware of your relationship with technology and learn how to make it work for you, instead of being a slave to it, it can actually do you a world of good.

TAKE CONTROL

Mindfulness is all about being present in the moment and free from distractions, which works against the attention-grabbing nature of our modern devices. The best starting point to achieving digital harmony is to assess your relationship with your tech. Consider how much time you spend using your phone, in front of the TV, and sitting at your workstation. If you find that most of your day involves screen time, try taking steps to reduce that.

While it is tempting, reaching for your phone as soon as you wake up might not be the best idea. The wake-up period can set your mood for the whole day, and stirring from your sleep only to check your phone to see doom and gloom in the news, for example, isn't going to put you on the path to a good mood. Instead, try

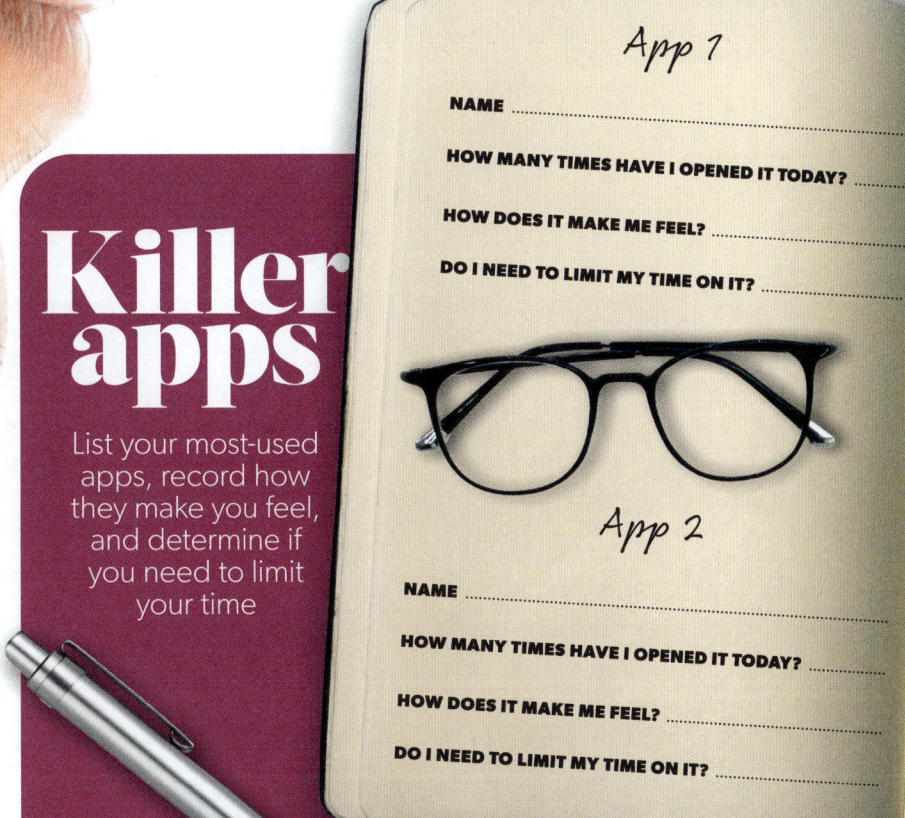

Killer apps

List your most-used apps, record how they make you feel, and determine if you need to limit your time

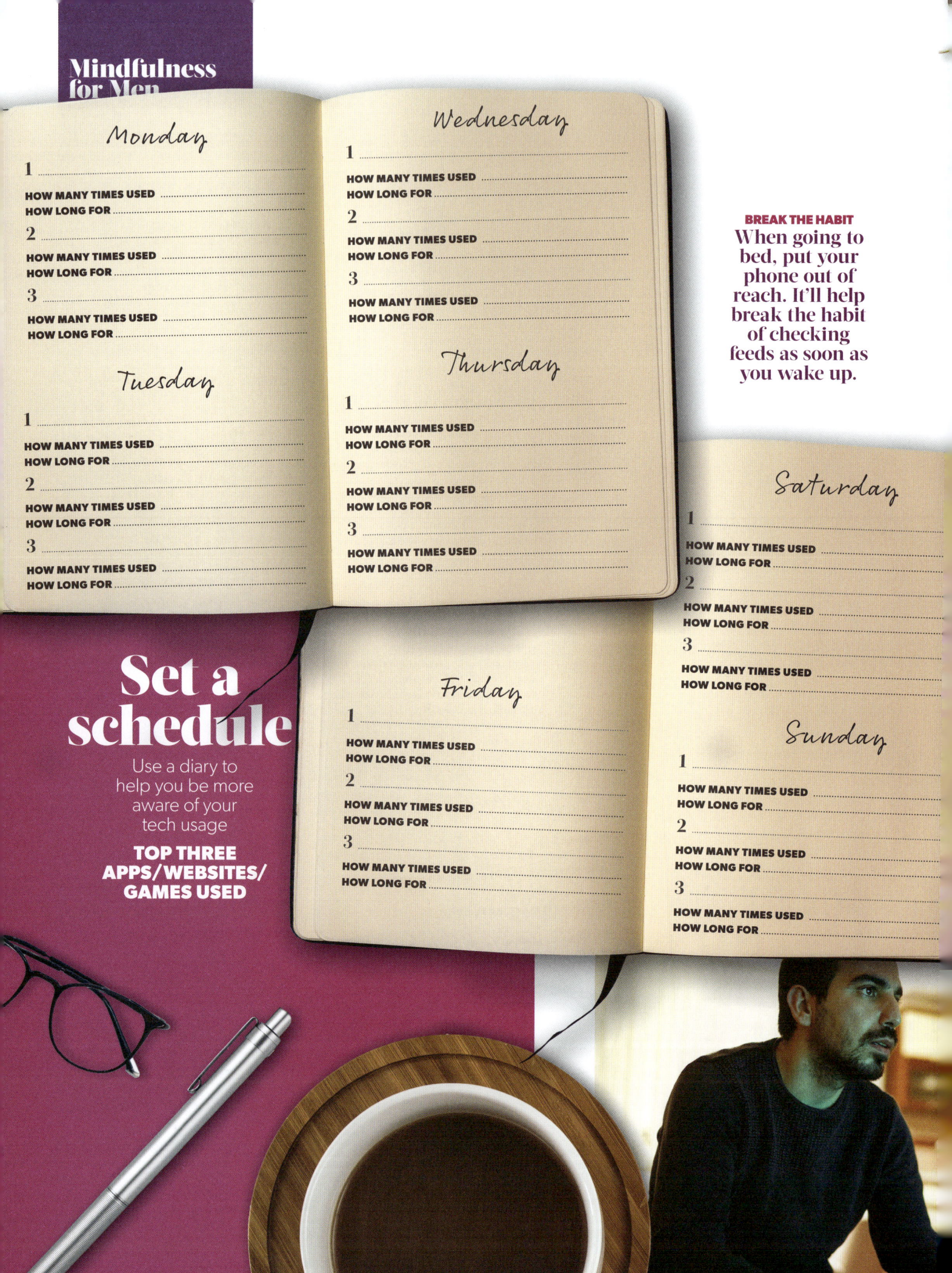

Mindfulness for Men

Monday

1 ....
HOW MANY TIMES USED ....
HOW LONG FOR ....

2 ....
HOW MANY TIMES USED ....
HOW LONG FOR ....

3 ....
HOW MANY TIMES USED ....
HOW LONG FOR ....

Tuesday

1 ....
HOW MANY TIMES USED ....
HOW LONG FOR ....

2 ....
HOW MANY TIMES USED ....
HOW LONG FOR ....

3 ....
HOW MANY TIMES USED ....
HOW LONG FOR ....

Wednesday

1 ....
HOW MANY TIMES USED ....
HOW LONG FOR ....

2 ....
HOW MANY TIMES USED ....
HOW LONG FOR ....

3 ....
HOW MANY TIMES USED ....
HOW LONG FOR ....

Thursday

1 ....
HOW MANY TIMES USED ....
HOW LONG FOR ....

2 ....
HOW MANY TIMES USED ....
HOW LONG FOR ....

3 ....
HOW MANY TIMES USED ....
HOW LONG FOR ....

Friday

1 ....
HOW MANY TIMES USED ....
HOW LONG FOR ....

2 ....
HOW MANY TIMES USED ....
HOW LONG FOR ....

3 ....
HOW MANY TIMES USED ....
HOW LONG FOR ....

Saturday

1 ....
HOW MANY TIMES USED ....
HOW LONG FOR ....

2 ....
HOW MANY TIMES USED ....
HOW LONG FOR ....

3 ....
HOW MANY TIMES USED ....
HOW LONG FOR ....

Sunday

1 ....
HOW MANY TIMES USED ....
HOW LONG FOR ....

2 ....
HOW MANY TIMES USED ....
HOW LONG FOR ....

3 ....
HOW MANY TIMES USED ....
HOW LONG FOR ....

BREAK THE HABIT
When going to bed, put your phone out of reach. It'll help break the habit of checking feeds as soon as you wake up.

Set a schedule

Use a diary to help you be more aware of your tech usage

TOP THREE APPS/WEBSITES/GAMES USED

Pulling the plug

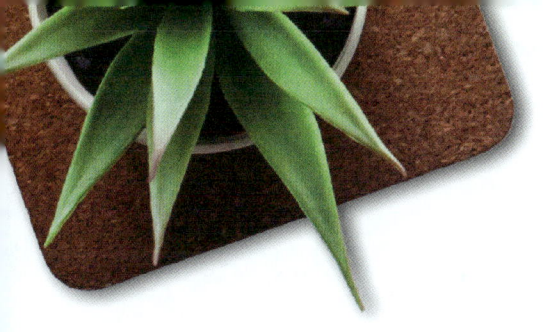

leaving your phone while you perform your morning activities. Give your mind the time it needs to stir from its sleep-addled stupor, and you will find that your mood might be lighter than when you wake up and tumble headfirst into a torrent of notifications.

If you find yourself using social media more than you'd like, and feel its grip over your attention is a bit *too* strong to break away from, it's not the end of the world. Your devices have useful features buried in their settings that will help monitor and limit your usage. For example, iPhones have 'Screen Time', which tracks how long you use certain apps and can limit access to them. Android devices have a similar feature called 'Digital Wellbeing', which helps you unplug from daily distractions.

GLOOM AND DOOMSCROLL
When viewing content, what you consume is as important as how much. While keeping abreast of current events and news is a good idea, it can be a downer. There's an unwritten rule in news writing: bad news sells, and this negativity bias takes over both the journalist choosing which stories to promote, as well as the reader choosing which stories to read.

It's extremely easy to fall into a spiral of doomscrolling, obsessively consuming one despair story to another. From overseas wars to cost-of-living crises and political clown shows, we're not short of negative news in the modern world, and exposing yourself to this black hole of bleakness will affect your mood. Additionally, you might switch from watching the news on TV to checking social media, only to see the people you follow are sharing similar negative stories, creating a self-sustaining maelstrom of misery.

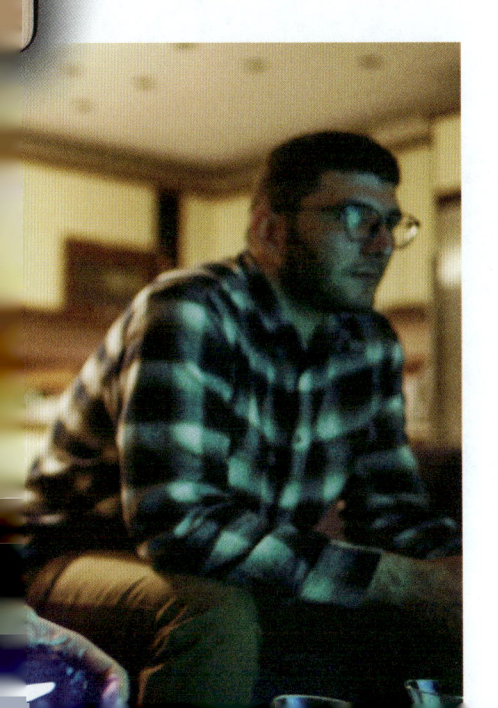

The remedy to this is easy to say but hard to implement: don't engage with it as much. Be more aware of when you check the news and your social feeds, and how long for. The more you're conscious of your usage, the easier it is to limit it. It's also worth turning off notifications for any news service or social media you use. You can also consider deleting any apps causing you grief, or at least bury them in a folder beyond your home screen so they're not easily accessible.

GAME-CHANGER
Modern technology is obviously not limited to that tiny black rectangle living inside your pocket. Playing video games such as FIFA, Fortnite or Call Of Duty is as commonplace as watching the latest must-see Netflix series, but these experiences can get addictive and will demand more and more of your time.

Premium battle passes and online ranked tables are all designed to keep you coming back, and it's vital to understand that. While unlocking awesome-looking aesthetics for your character or progressing from gold to platinum tiers is an undeniable rush, remember that it's *you* playing the game, and make sure that the game doesn't play you.

By all means, incorporate gaming into your daily routine, but commit to a few hours a day and not an entire evening. High-stakes showdowns with other players online are compelling but also stressful: if you're often using this to unwind after a high-pressure workday, you'll run yourself ragged.

A FORCE FOR GOOD
While tech can hinder a mindful lifestyle, it can also help. A clear benefit of technology with mindfulness is the wealth of apps available. The likes of Headspace, Calm, Loóna, and more help cultivate a peaceful state of mind by playing soothing music and provide calming breathing exercises that help you focus and soothe anxiety or stress. You can also harness gaming as a mindfulness exercise. Games like Tetris Effect, Minecraft and Journey are meditative experiences where you can let pleasant sights and sounds wash over you while completing the relaxing objectives they present.

Technology is a powerful tool at our disposal, however it can burn you out. That said, if you can establish boundaries and use its power to aid you, it's an almighty means to help you improve your mindfulness journey. What's most exciting is that it's constantly evolving, with enterprising developers finding new ways to harness this modern wonder to enhance our lives.

Peace of mind
Want to use technology to improve mindfulness? Try these examples…

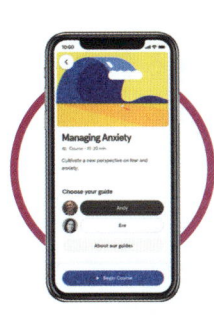

HEADSPACE
For those who want to incorporate meditation in a non-intimidating way, try Headspace. None of the mindfulness or meditation exercises last longer than 30 minutes, making them easy to squeeze into your day. You'll eventually have to pay for a subscription, but you can try before you buy with a free trial.

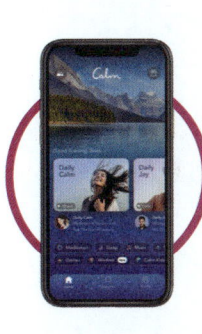

CALM
Featuring celebrity-led exercises from the likes of LeBron James and Matthew McConaughey, Calm is packed with content that will help dispel stress. It's a versatile platform, offering meditation as well as sleep and children-focused exercises. As is the case with Headspace, there's a free trial to test out the premium version.

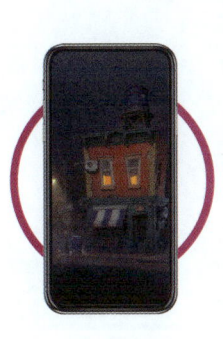

LOÓNA
If your sleep is affected by anxiety and stress, Loóna is worth a look. It's unique in that it presents you with 'Sleepscapes', dioramas that you colour in while a narrator describes a calming story to soothing music that helps put you at ease. There are short, free exercises you can try, and the full version unlocks full 20-minute Sleepscapes, stories and music you can drift off to.

Mindfulness for Men

SLEEP BETTER

Clearing the mind

The brain is a power-hungry organ; it makes up only 2% of the total mass of the body, but it uses an enormous 25% of the total energy supply. The question is, how does it get rid of waste? The Nedergaard Lab at the University of Rochester in New York thinks sleep might be a time to clean the brain. The rest of the body relies on the lymphatic drainage system to help remove waste products, but the brain is a protected area, and these vessels do not extend upward into the head. Instead, your central nervous system is bathed in a clear liquid called cerebrospinal fluid (CSF), into which waste can be dissolved for removal. During the day, it remains on the outside, but the lab's research has shown that during sleep, gaps open up between brain cells and the fluid rushes in, following paths along the outside of blood vessels, sweeping through every corner of the brain and helping to clear out toxic molecules.

Sleep better

What is sleep, why is it so important to us, and what happens when we don't get enough?

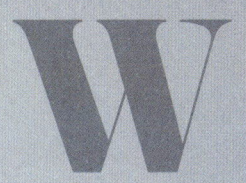

We spend around a third of our lives sleeping; it is vital to our survival, but despite years of research, scientists still aren't entirely sure why we do it. The urge to sleep is all-consuming, and if we are deprived of it, we will eventually slip into slumber even if the situation is life-threatening.

Sleep is common to mammals, birds and reptiles, and has been conserved through evolution, even though it prevents us from performing tasks such as eating, reproducing and raising young. It is as important as food for keeping us alive; without it, rats will die within two or three weeks – the same amount of time it takes to die of starvation.

There have been many theories about why we sleep, from a way to rest after the day's activities or a method for saving energy, to simply a way to fill time until we can be doing something useful, but all of these ideas are flawed. The body repairs itself just as well when we sit quietly – we only save around 100 calories a night by sleeping, and we wouldn't need to catch up on sleep during the day if it were just to fill empty time at night.

One of the major problems with sleep deprivation is a resulting decline in cognitive ability; our brains just don't work properly without sleep. We struggle with memory, learning, planning and reasoning. A lack of sleep can have severe effects on our performance, ranging from irritability and low mood, through to an increased risk of heart disease and a higher number of road traffic accidents.

Sleep can be divided into two broad stages: non-rapid eye movement (NREM), and rapid eye movement (REM) sleep. The vast majority of our sleep (around 75 to 80%) is NREM, characterised by electrical patterns in the brain known as 'sleep spindles' and high, slow delta waves. This is the time we sleep the deepest. Without NREM sleep, our ability to form declarative memories, such as learning to associate pairs of words, can be seriously impaired; deep sleep is important for transferring short-term memories into long-term storage. Deep sleep is also the time of peak growth hormone release in the body, which is important for cell reproduction and repair.

The purpose of REM sleep is unclear; the effects of REM sleep deprivation are less severe than NREM deprivation, and for the first two weeks humans report little in the way of ill effects. REM sleep is the period during the night when we have our most vivid dreams, but people dream during both NREM and REM sleep. During NREM sleep, dreams tend to be more concept-based, whereas during REM sleep dreams are more vivid and emotional.

Some scientists argue that REM sleep allows our brains a safe place to practise dealing with our emotions that we might not encounter during our daily lives. Others think that it might be a way to unlearn memories, or to process unwanted feelings or emotions. Each of these ideas has its flaws, and no one knows the real answer.

Over the next few pages we will delve into the science of sleep and attempt to make sense of the mysteries of the sleeping brain.

THE CYCLE

During the night, you cycle through five separate stages of sleep every 90 to 110 minutes

The five stages of sleep can be distinguished by changes in the electrical activity in your brain, measured by electroencephalogram (EEG). The first stage begins with drowsiness as you drift in and out of consciousness, and is followed by light sleep and then by two stages of deep sleep. Your brain activity starts to slow down; your breathing, heart rate and temperature drop; and you become progressively more difficult to wake up. Finally, your brain perks up again, resuming activity that looks much more like wakefulness, and you enter rapid eye movement (REM) sleep, the time that your most vivid dreams occur. This cycle happens several times throughout the night, and each time, the period of REM sleep grows longer.

Stages of sleep

Not all sleep is the same; there are five separate stages, divided up by brain activity

1. Drowsiness

During the first stage of sleep, you are just drifting off; your eyelids are heavy and your head starts to drop. During this drowsy period, you are easily awoken and your brain is still quite active. The electrical activity on an electroencephalogram (EEG) monitor starts to slow down, and the cortical waves become taller and spikier. As the sleep cycle repeats during the night, you re-enter this drowsy half-awake, half-asleep stage.

2. Light sleep

After a few minutes, your brain activity slows further, and you descend into light sleep. On the EEG monitor, this stage is characterised by further slowing in the waves with an increase in their size, and short one or two-second bursts of activity known as 'sleep spindles'. By the time you are in the second phase of sleep, your eyes stop moving, but you can still be woken quite easily.

3. Moderate sleep

As you start to enter this stage, your sleep spindles stop, showing that your brain has entered moderate sleep. This is then followed by deep sleep. The trace on the EEG slows still further as your brain produces delta waves with occasional spikes of smaller faster waves in between. As you progress through stage-three sleep, you become much more difficult to wake up.

4. Deep sleep

There is some debate as to whether sleep stages three and four are really separate, or whether they are part of the same phase of sleep. Stage four is the deepest stage, and during this time, you are extremely hard to wake. The EEG shows tall, slow waves known as delta waves, your muscles relax, and your breathing becomes slow and rhythmic, which can lead to snoring.

5. REM sleep

After deep sleep, your brain starts to perk up and its electrical activity starts to resemble the waking brain. This is the period of the night when most dreams happen. Your muscles are temporarily paralysed, and your eyes dart back and forth, giving this stage its name, rapid eye movement (REM) sleep. You cycle through the stages of sleep about every 90 minutes, experiencing between three and five dream periods each night.

How much time do you spend in each sleep stage?

- 30% OTHER STAGES
- 20% REM SLEEP
- 50% STAGE 2 SLEEP

Sleep better

DREAMING VERSUS DEEP SLEEP

FIRST CYCLE | SECOND CYCLE | THIRD CYCLE | FOURTH CYCLE | FIFTH CYCLE

WAKE
REM
STAGE 1
STAGE 2
STAGE 3
STAGE 4

■ DEEP SLEEP   DREAMING (REM)

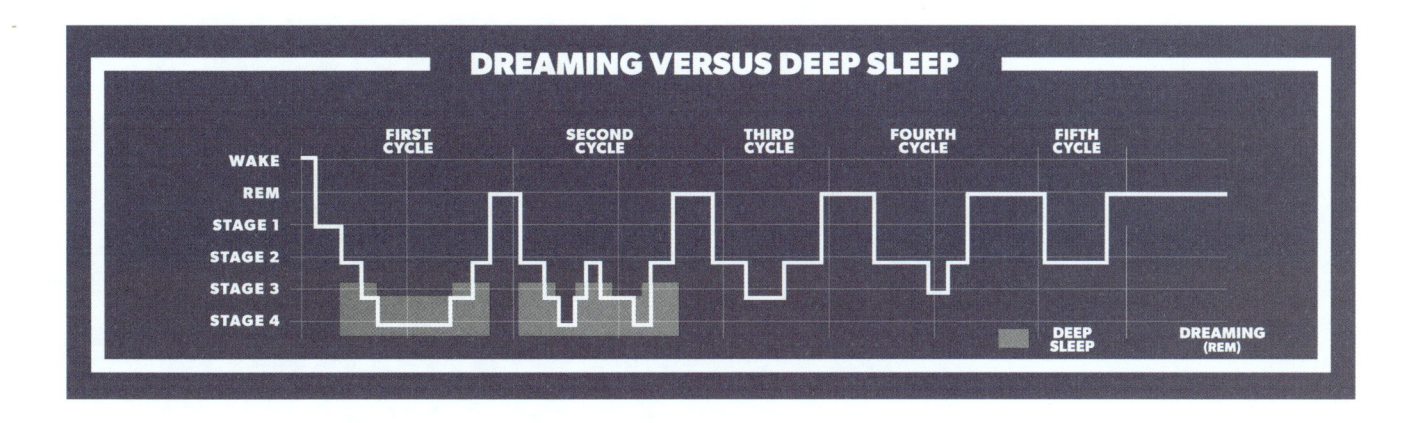

How to get a good night's sleep

Understanding your biological clock is the key to a healthy night's sleep

Your body is driven by an internal circadian master clock known as the suprachiasmatic nucleus, which is set on a time scale of roughly 24 hours and influenced by light. Disruptions in light exposure can play havoc with your sleep, so it is important to ensure that your bedroom is as dark as possible. Many electronic devices produce enough light to reset your biological clock, and using backlit screens late at night can confuse your brain, preventing the production of melatonin and delaying your sleep.

Another important factor in a good night's sleep is winding down before bed. Stimulants like caffeine and nicotine keep your brain alert and can seriously disrupt your sleep, and even depressants like alcohol can have a negative effect; even though it calms the brain, it interferes with normal sleep cycles, preventing proper deep and REM sleep.

BRAIN ACTIVITY

WIDE AWAKE
The red areas in this scan show areas of activity in the waking human brain, while the blue areas represent areas of inactivity in the brain.

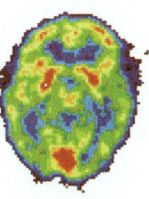

REM (DREAM) SLEEP
When the brain is dreaming, it is very active, showing similar red patterns of activity to the waking brain.

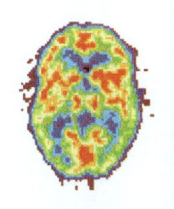

SLEEP DEPRIVATION
The sleep-deprived brain looks similar to the brain during NREM sleep, showing patterns of inactivity in the brain.

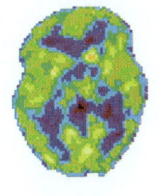

DEEP SLEEP
During the later stages of NREM sleep, the brain is less active, shown here by the cool blue and purple colours that dominate the scan.

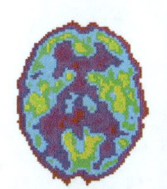

LIGHT SLEEP
The first stages of NREM sleep, the brain is less active than when awake, but you remain alert and easy to wake up.

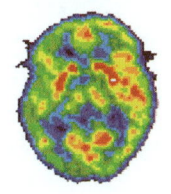

NREM SLEEP
As you descend through the four stages of NREM sleep, your brain becomes progressively less active than before.

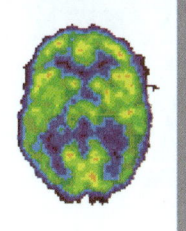

THE DANGERS OF SLEEP DEPRIVATION

IMPAIRED JUDGEMENT
Sleep deprivation impacts your visual working memory, as well as affecting your emotional intelligence, behaviour and ability to manage stress.

WEIGHT GAIN
Lack of sleep affects appetite-regulating hormones. Levels of the hormone that tells you how much stored fat you have drop, and hunger hormones rise.

RAISED BLOOD PRESSURE
Poor sleep can raise blood pressure, and in the long term is associated with an increased risk of diseases such as coronary heart disease and stroke.

INCREASED ACCIDENTS
It's estimated that 100,000 road accidents each year in the US result from driver fatigue, and over a third of drivers have admitted to falling asleep at the wheel.

MOOD DISORDERS
Mental health problems are linked to poor sleep, and deprivation can play havoc with the brain, causing symptoms of depression, anxiety and mania.

HALLUCINATIONS
Severe sleep deprivation can lead to hallucinations. In rare cases it can even lead to temporary psychosis or symptoms that resemble paranoid schizophrenia.

Mindfulness for Men

Gratitude is a magical tool that we should all be tapping into more frequently. You'll soon begin to see there are so many reasons to be grateful – you just have to allow yourself the time to notice them

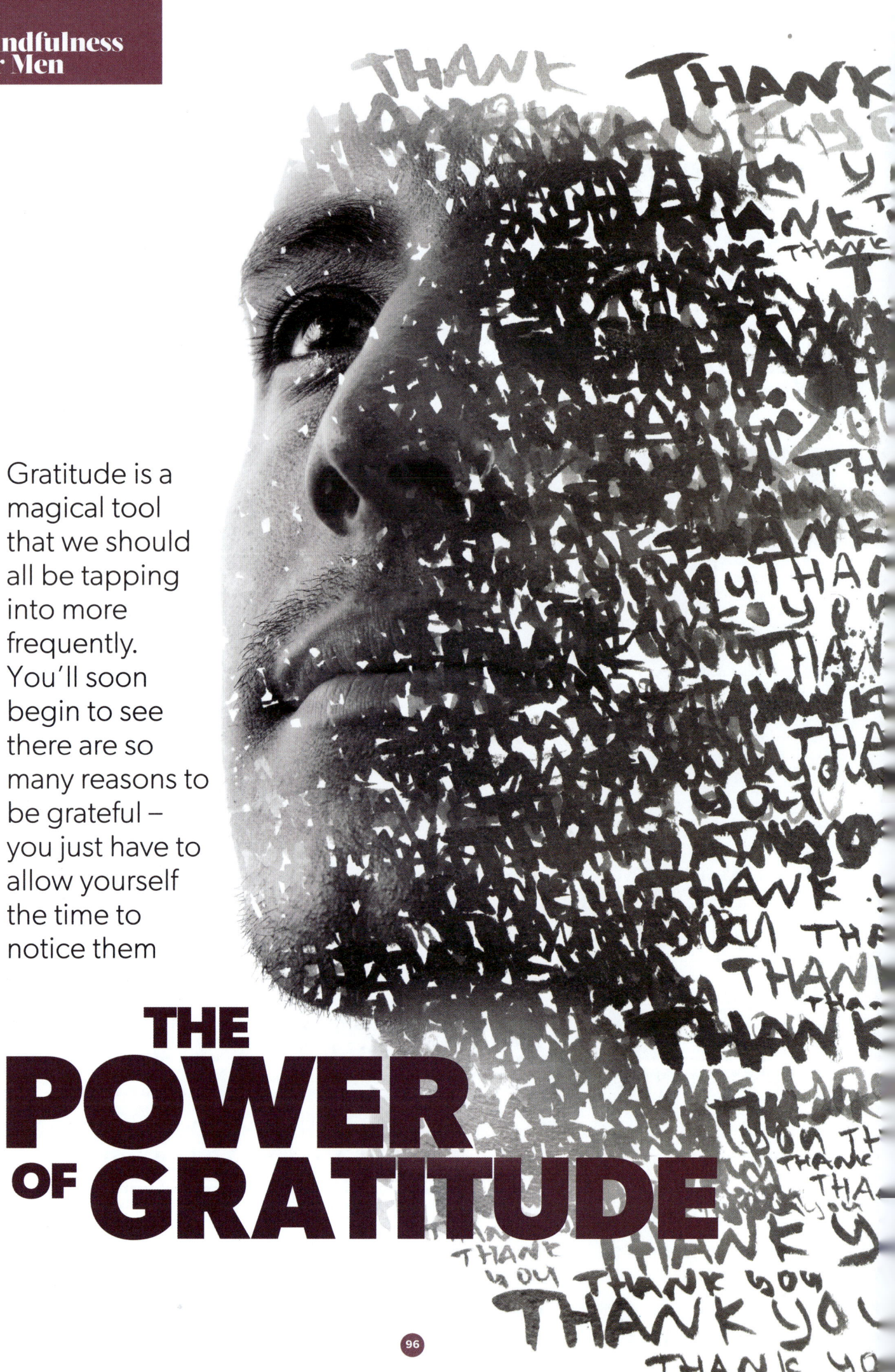

THE POWER OF GRATITUDE

The power of gratitude

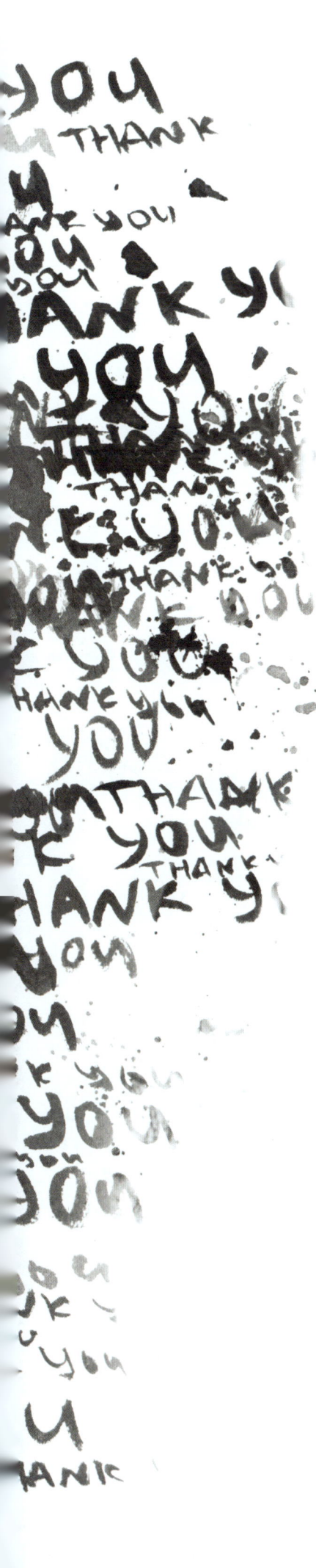

How many times have you found something irritating today? How many times have you focused on the negative things that have happened? Now how many times have you made a mental note of something positive that happened? We are all guilty of focusing on life's tiny burdens instead of remaining mindful of our blessings and how lucky we are to be alive. For many years, gratitude has played an important part in a lot of religious and spiritual practices as a way of connecting us to the present moment and reaffirming how precious life can be. Whether you believe in destiny or not, sometimes it might feel as though we have little control over which direction our lives are going. But gratitude teaches us that we have a choice about what we focus our attention on. By making time to write gratitude lists, we gain control over our minds, forcing ourselves to focus on the good rather than the bad.

According to author Eckhart Tolle, "the mind exists in a state of 'not enough' and so [it] is always greedy for more." Our minds are continuously in overdrive, striving for the next best thing – whether that's a new car, a new pair of shoes or the latest tech device. We are always trying to better ourselves in one way or another. In doing so, we might have become a bit lost, and forgotten what truly makes us content. But hope is not lost just yet. What we can all be doing more of is stopping to appreciate what we already have around us. In the modern, technology-filled world, our minds are being stimulated more than ever, and sometimes this can mean that we find ourselves turning to consumerism for an instant 'fix' to enrich our lives. In doing so, we bypass the most simple fact – that life is full to the brim of moments of joy that money cannot buy. Gratitude teaches us to stop, pause and reflect on our own lives, and be thankful for all that we have. Gratitude also steers our attention away from negativity and instead focuses on the hidden treasures that can be found in the simple pleasures of life.

Love thy neighbour
Make a list of random acts of kindness people have shown you.

WHY IS GRATITUDE IMPORTANT IN THE MODERN WORLD?
Over the course of the last 100 years, we have forgotten how to find pleasure in the everyday things in life. Through no fault of our own, modern life has become increasingly more complicated, stressful and busy, which is why it's more important than ever for us to strip everything back and remind ourselves of what truly gives us purpose, makes us tick and brings a smile to our faces. Life can become crazy from time to time, with many of us struggling to manage our own schedules efficiently and find balance between our professional and personal lives. It is here in the humdrum that some of us may have lost sight of what is actually important to us. Take a moment now and think about your typical day. Do you frequently reach the evening wondering 'where did the day go?' Are you pausing to appreciate the great moments that you have experienced over the course of the day? Did you make a note of them? If you answered no to the latter questions, then the good news is you've come to the right place. It's time

Mindfulness for Men

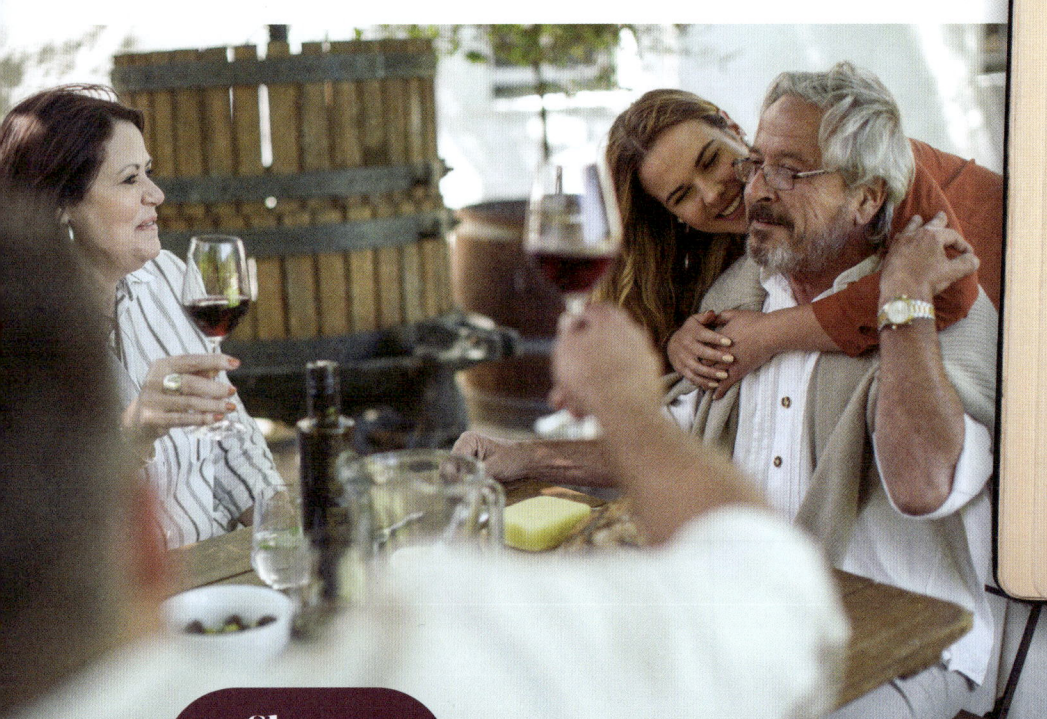

My favourite things

Think about three physical possessions you're grateful for and why.

1 ....
....
....
....

Share the love

As we go through life, we might forget how important some of the key people in our lives truly are. You might find when writing on these pages that you are frequently grateful for people. Most of us have a small support network of friends and family members who continuously show up for us. It's more important than ever that we let these people know how invaluable they are to our mental health and overall happiness, so don't hesitate to tell them and show them some love.

to start appreciating everything life has to offer.

THE POWER OF PAUSING, SLOWING DOWN AND LIVING IN THE PRESENT MOMENT

When life becomes busy and hectic, it can be very easy to live our lives on autopilot, but in doing so we miss all the best bits. This is where gratitude becomes invaluable, as it helps to redirect us when we feel a bit lost. Whenever we're overwhelmed or feeling down, gratitude forces us to concentrate on the here and now, and remind ourselves of life's simple pleasures. Using a gratitude journal will provide you with a safe space to reflect from time to time, enabling you to focus on the present moment and appreciate the small things that spark contentment in your life. Allowing yourself this time for contemplation every now and again lets you shine a light on all of the positive elements in your life – even when it might feel like there aren't any. You'll soon find there is a lot more to be grateful for than you first thought.

GRATITUDE COMES IN ALL SHAPES AND SIZES

We all have different things that we are grateful for day to day. Many people would consider similar themes: family, friends, health, love and having a place to call home. These are all valid, of course, but why specifically are we grateful for them? Perhaps you are struggling to find everyday things to be grateful for. Maybe

Above: It's so important to let the people you love and appreciate know how much you value them

you're finding it hard to pinpoint exactly what made you happy today. These are all common feelings.

The good news is that you are not alone – we all have good days and bad days. Sometimes our happiest moments on the tough days are as simple as crawling into bed after a long day at work, or enjoying a cup of tea in the morning. Life is complicated enough – you don't need to make things harder for yourself by trying to think of interesting anecdotes or original content for each entry. Let's strip everything back and get down to the basic elements of your life because, more often than not, the simple things in life are the things that make us the happiest.

THE NEWFOUND JOY OF SIMPLE THINGS

One of the many benefits of gratitude is its ability to teach us how to slow down in our fast-paced lives. A big problem with our constant consumption of entertainment and our over-stimulation in the digital world is that we are forgetting how to stop and notice the small things. We are unintentionally living on fast forward and not acknowledging how beautiful our lives are.

When you become more mindful of gratitude, you might find that you begin to feel grateful for something that you wouldn't have necessarily noticed before. Some of these small pleasures could be stopping and appreciating the wonderful flavours in your dinner, that cuddle with

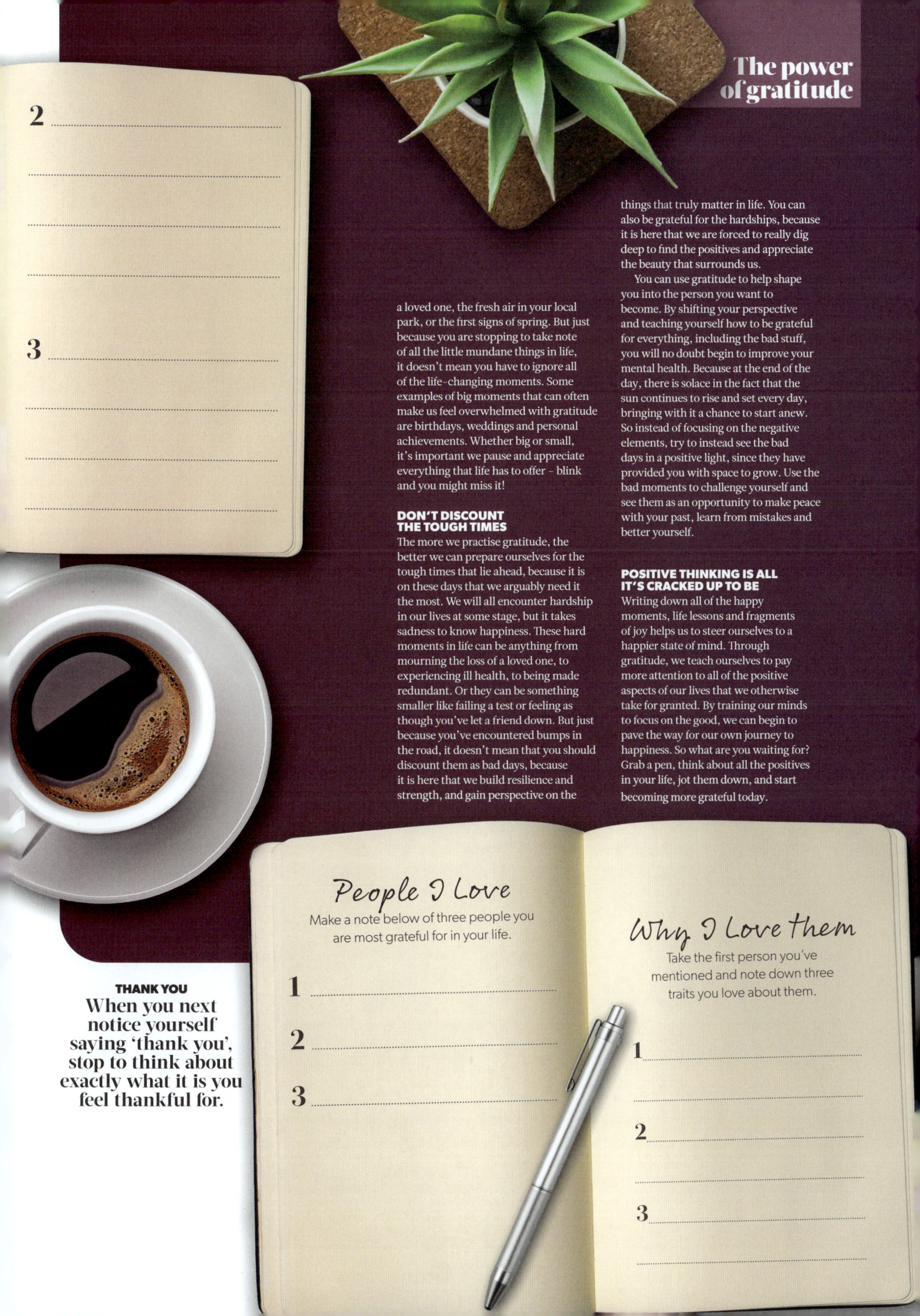

The power of gratitude

a loved one, the fresh air in your local park, or the first signs of spring. But just because you are stopping to take note of all the little mundane things in life, it doesn't mean you have to ignore all of the life-changing moments. Some examples of big moments that can often make us feel overwhelmed with gratitude are birthdays, weddings and personal achievements. Whether big or small, it's important we pause and appreciate everything that life has to offer – blink and you might miss it!

DON'T DISCOUNT THE TOUGH TIMES

The more we practise gratitude, the better we can prepare ourselves for the tough times that lie ahead, because it is on these days that we arguably need it the most. We will all encounter hardship in our lives at some stage, but it takes sadness to know happiness. These hard moments in life can be anything from mourning the loss of a loved one, to experiencing ill health, to being made redundant. Or they can be something smaller like failing a test or feeling as though you've let a friend down. But just because you've encountered bumps in the road, it doesn't mean that you should discount them as bad days, because it is here that we build resilience and strength, and gain perspective on the things that truly matter in life. You can also be grateful for the hardships, because it is here that we are forced to really dig deep to find the positives and appreciate the beauty that surrounds us.

You can use gratitude to help shape you into the person you want to become. By shifting your perspective and teaching yourself how to be grateful for everything, including the bad stuff, you will no doubt begin to improve your mental health. Because at the end of the day, there is solace in the fact that the sun continues to rise and set every day, bringing with it a chance to start anew. So instead of focusing on the negative elements, try to instead see the bad days in a positive light, since they have provided you with space to grow. Use the bad moments to challenge yourself and see them as an opportunity to make peace with your past, learn from mistakes and better yourself.

POSITIVE THINKING IS ALL IT'S CRACKED UP TO BE

Writing down all of the happy moments, life lessons and fragments of joy helps us to steer ourselves to a happier state of mind. Through gratitude, we teach ourselves to pay more attention to all of the positive aspects of our lives that we otherwise take for granted. By training our minds to focus on the good, we can begin to pave the way for our own journey to happiness. So what are you waiting for? Grab a pen, think about all the positives in your life, jot them down, and start becoming more grateful today.

THANK YOU
When you next notice yourself saying 'thank you', stop to think about exactly what it is you feel thankful for.

People I Love
Make a note below of three people you are most grateful for in your life.

1 ....
2 ....
3 ....

Why I Love Them
Take the first person you've mentioned and note down three traits you love about them.

1 ....
2 ....
3 ....

Mindfulness for Men

MAKE A HABIT, BREAK A HABIT

Our brains never forget old habits (this is why we can always ride a bike, even if it's been years since we were last on one), but we do favour new habits over old ones

Habits are, essentially, shortcuts for your brain. They are efficient, because they mean you can automate actions while your brain focuses on other things. Whether you know it or not, you've been training yourself to do certain tasks by rote and in response to cues.

However, your brain doesn't know the difference, chemically, between a 'good' habit and one that is 'bad' (like biting fingernails or a social media addiction). 'Pleasure-based habits' encourage the release of dopamine (our brain's happy chemical), and since we crave dopamine, we are rewarded to do the habit again. We can use mindfulness to change the habits we consider bad and help ourselves stick to the good habits we want to foster.

BREAKING BAD HABITS
Work on becoming more mindful when taking part in your habits (whether 'good' or 'bad'). How do they make you feel in yourself? You will find that, at its most basic, our brains follow a pattern – trigger, behaviour, reward. So we can use mindfulness to dig a little deeper into the 'trigger' part of the pattern and we can turn off the automatic part of a habit. We can start by asking ourselves 'Why?' when a bad habit rears its ugly head. Breathe fully to remind yourself to be present, be kind to yourself, and if you find your mind wandering, or if you talk to yourself unkindly, bring yourself back to the task at hand with kindness; you're not looking to beat yourself up, but to better understand yourself. Why and what are you feeling when you reach for a certain habit (pattern of behaviour)? Is it comfort you're looking for? How could you re-

Make a habit, break a habit

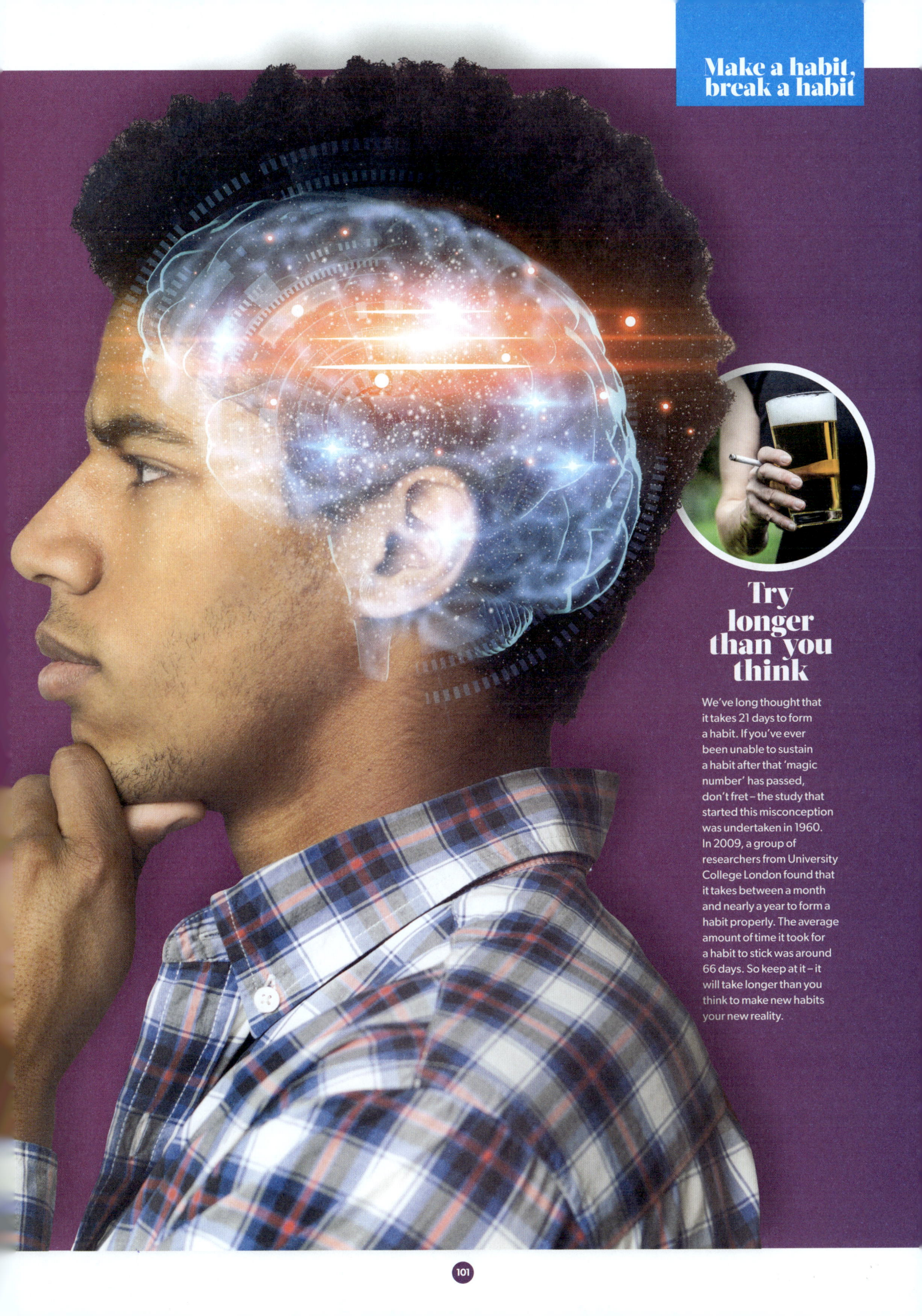

Try longer than you think

We've long thought that it takes 21 days to form a habit. If you've ever been unable to sustain a habit after that 'magic number' has passed, don't fret – the study that started this misconception was undertaken in 1960. In 2009, a group of researchers from University College London found that it takes between a month and nearly a year to form a habit properly. The average amount of time it took for a habit to stick was around 66 days. So keep at it – it will take longer than you think to make new habits your new reality.

Mindfulness for Men

Finding it hard?

While it can take between 18 to 250 days to form a new habit, there is a group of people for whom it may feel even more difficult. Many people are 'habit resistant'. It's important to be kind to yourself if you feel like this may be you. Changing behaviours is tricky, especially if you're beginning a habit that is hard work to stick to, like a difficult exercise, or trying to stop a 'bad' habit.

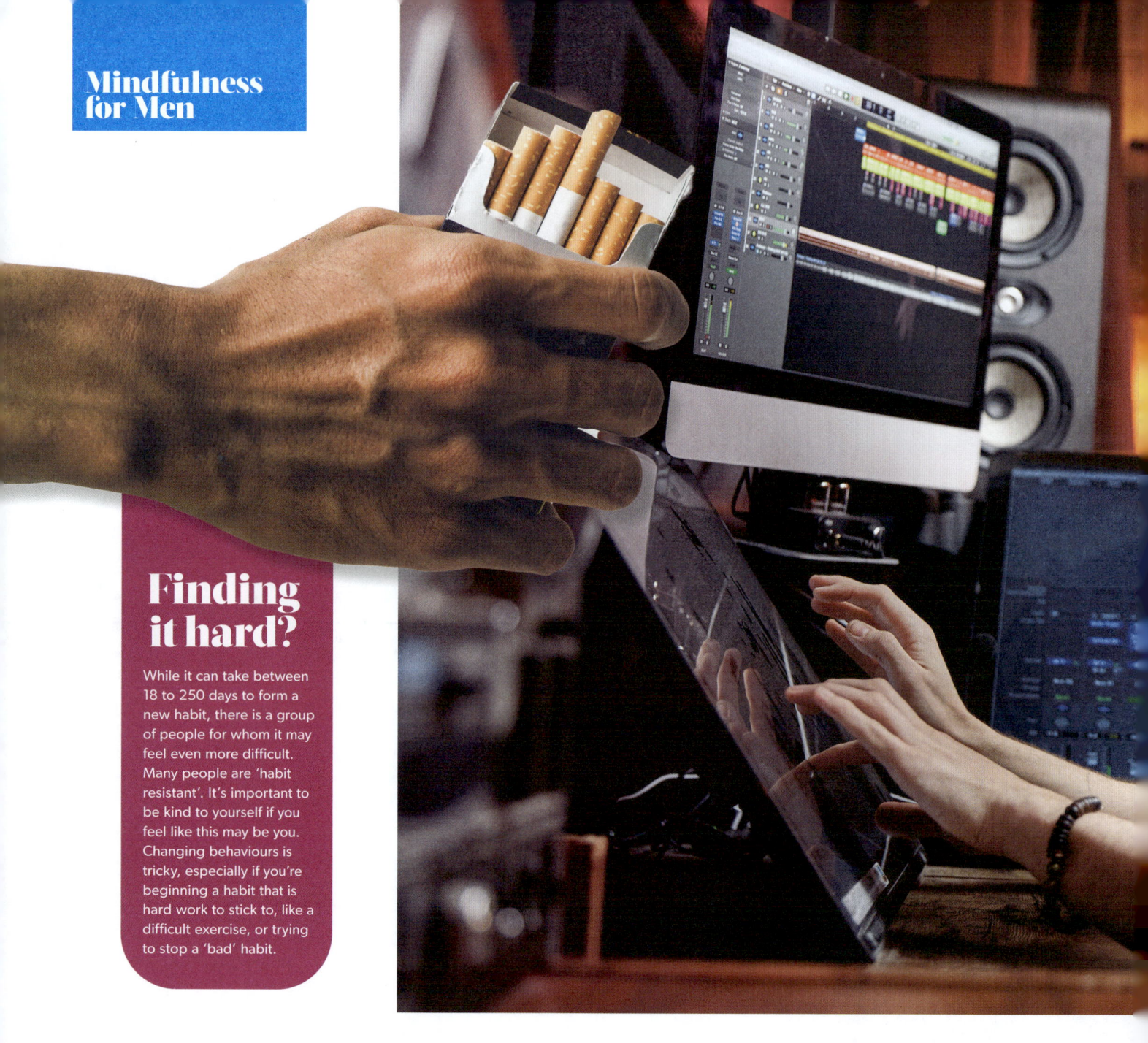

MINDFUL HABITS

There are reams and reams of positive habits that you can take up, whether to improve your day-to-day or to replace the bad habits you've fostered. There is also a vast array of mindful habits to adopt. Remember to start slowly and not rush to adopt all the mindful habits at once – that would only serve to set you up to fail, and feelings of failure are not what we're looking to cultivate.

Divide your habits into four areas.

1. Physical: feel your environment, breathe deeply, be mindful when eating.

2. Emotional: practise being grateful, cry if you need to.

3. Intellectual: listen to your intuition, speak kindly to yourself and others.

4. Creative: read, when you create (food/art/anything), take note of the sensations you experience.

Remember a key component of mindfulness is to live in the here and now. Be aware of the real nature of what you are experiencing. Work on fully living and enjoying your new habits. Be kind to yourself and remember that life changes quickly – what works for you one month might not work a few months later.

WRITE IT DOWN!

A key technique in helping ourselves stick to the new habit is to journal them. Write your intention down – what are you looking to achieve and why? The 'why' can help you if you find a habit isn't sticking – what's your end goal? Remind yourself of it mindfully. Habit trackers are also incredibly helpful in journalling good habits – or even the bad! Instead of noting a long list of 'things I must remember to do', make a chart with the date at the top or side and your list of 'to dos' on the other; you can then colour them in if you hit your habit (or colour in if you break a habit that day). Take pleasure in filling out your tracker; keep an eye on how your mood changes when you complete a full row of colours. Use your favourite colours or change them every month to keep it interesting visually.

IF AND WHEN YOU FAIL

There are many strategies you can use if you fail at sticking to a habit; and you will – you're only human! Our habits can be broken down by difficulty level, and it's important to be kind to yourself. Remember one day missed doesn't matter; work on not missing two days.

Make a habit, break a habit

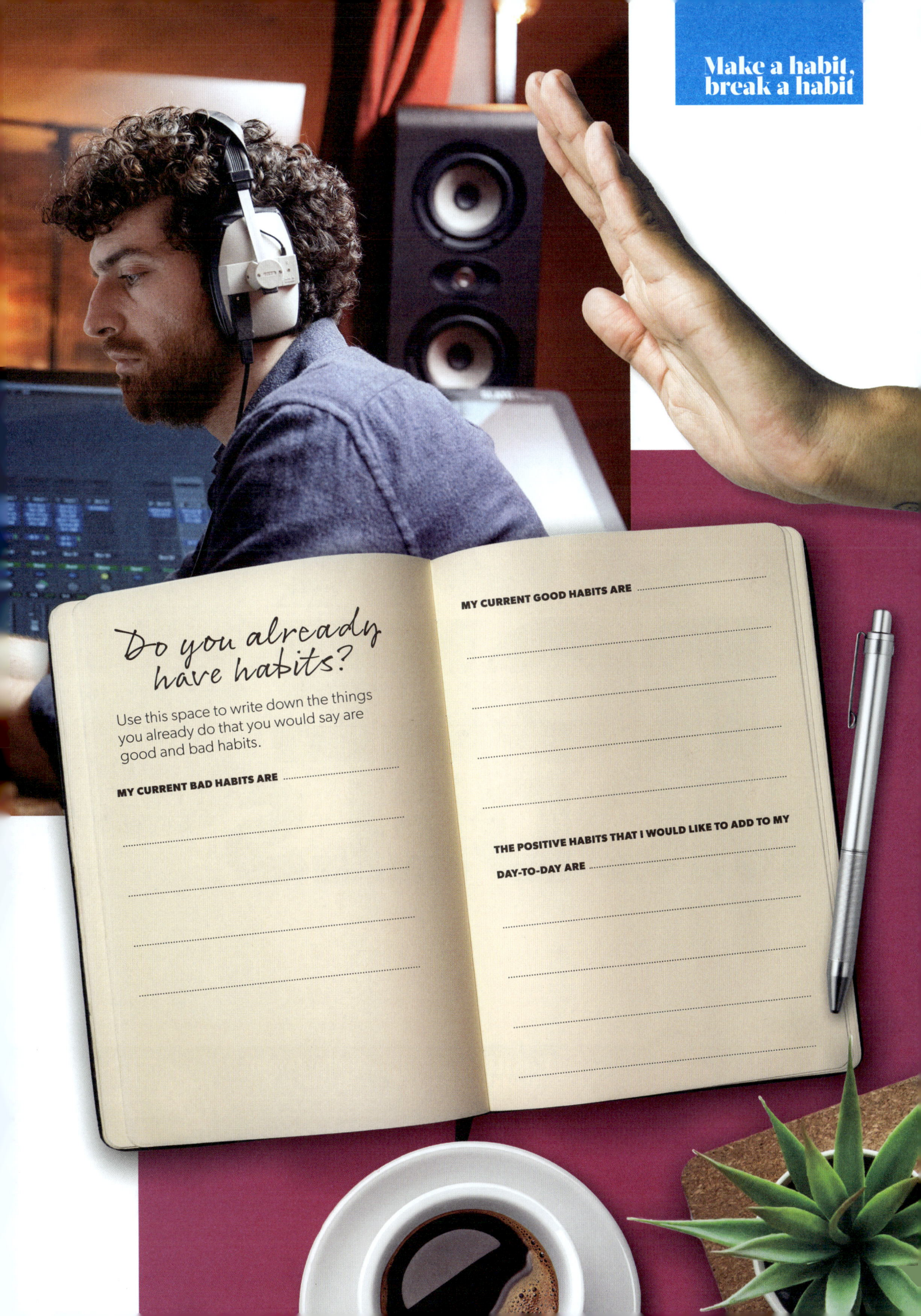

Do you already have habits?

Use this space to write down the things you already do that you would say are good and bad habits.

MY CURRENT BAD HABITS ARE ....
....
....
....
....

MY CURRENT GOOD HABITS ARE ....
....
....
....
....

THE POSITIVE HABITS THAT I WOULD LIKE TO ADD TO MY DAY-TO-DAY ARE ....
....
....
....
....

Mindfulness for Men

Take positive steps to becoming a better person by learning valuable lessons from those around you

KNOWING YOUR ROLE MODELS

Positive notes

What makes a good role model can be specific to your own needs, however, these following traits should have universal appeal

EMPATHY SAVANT
A person who is understanding, patient and a good listener is an ideal candidate for a role model. Encouraging others to speak up about what's troubling them as well as what's making them feel good is important.

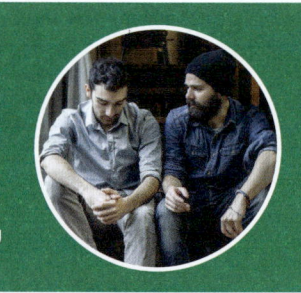

HOW TO BE A ROLE MODEL

Be confident in your abilities but also willing to address mistakes: admitting an error is not a sign of weakness.

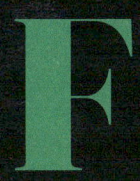

F rom an early age, we often look up to aspiring people around us. These can be parents or other family members, teachers, friends or figures from the wider world – even from fiction. These role models come into our lives in myriad ways, and looking to them as guiding stars of morality, physical fitness and mental acuity is highly beneficial to our development in our formative years.

But why stop there? Growing up is a journey, one that never ends, and having waypoints to guide us on this road will help prevent us straying from the path and away from the people we aspire to be. In turn, a positive outlook on internal growth and a willingness to better yourself by having a role model can inspire others. Eventually, *you* could become a role model to your peers, family and wider community.

REMEMBER YOUR ROLE MODELS
Think back to who your role models were when you were younger. Remembering their traits, what you admired about them, and what you feel about them today as an adult is a beneficial mindfulness exercise. Consider whether your values still align with them and if you successfully embraced their positive traits into your own life. They could still serve as a role model to you now.

While it is good to look back, it's also critical to look at the present as well as the future. Ask yourself, who are your role models now? If you have one, what is it about them that inspires you to learn from them? Try writing down or mentally planning steps you could take to incorporate their positive traits into your life. If possible, consider talking to them and exploring the possibilities of them helping you along the way.

If you don't believe you have any role models as an adult, think about why that is. Once you start thinking of people, personalities and characters you enjoy watching or being around, you might find you have a few without realising it.

WHAT MAKES A GOOD ROLE MODEL
Often, people fall into the trap of measuring a person's success as criteria for being a good role model. However, some celebrities or businesspeople possess questionable qualities that lead them to have a following that they might not necessarily have earned.

While success can emphasise positive traits, like the drive to do your best, you would do well to do your homework when determining role model candidates. Blindly following the latest eccentric business mogul or magnetic YouTube superstar could end up burning you in the long run. Consider looking up to people who are selfless and accepting of others, who seek to add value to the world around them and who strive to overcome obstacles while elevating others to do the same.

It can be easier than you think to find those qualities in the people you see in the media and those around you. Terry Crews, for example, is a highly driven individual who uses his platform to encourage men to open up about their problems. Marcus Rashford displays compassion for those less fortunate than him, and pressured the UK government to reverse a decision regarding free school meals. And it's hard not to be inspired by the love David Attenborough displays for our planet and its wildlife by tirelessly

EQUALITY CHAMPION
Someone who challenges gender roles in a positive way is a person worth following. A parent who doesn't hesitate to share the burden of household or childcare chores, or a peer who speaks up for those who need a helping hand are perfect role models.

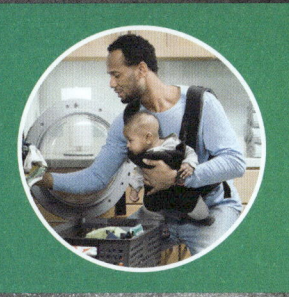

SELF-CARE SUPERSTAR
How can you help others get their life together if you can't look after yourself? Look towards individuals who strive to keep fit both mentally and physically – and aren't afraid to ask for a helping hand – for inspiration in your own life.

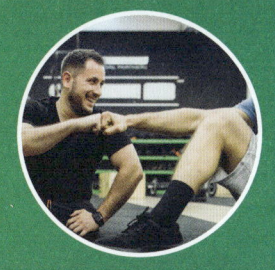

My top 10
Write down who you admire most in life.

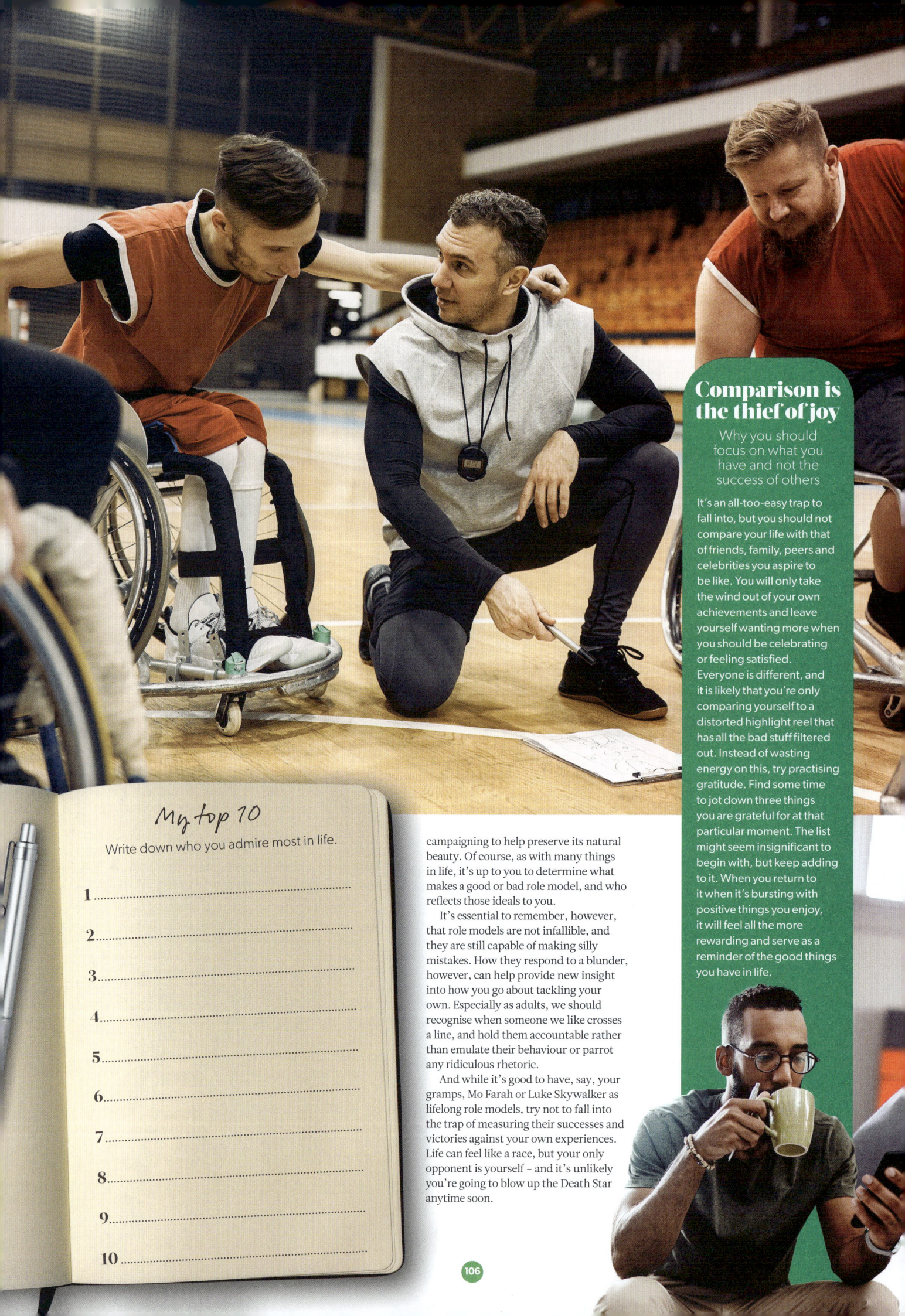

1. ....
2. ....
3. ....
4. ....
5. ....
6. ....
7. ....
8. ....
9. ....
10. ....

campaigning to help preserve its natural beauty. Of course, as with many things in life, it's up to you to determine what makes a good or bad role model, and who reflects those ideals to you.

It's essential to remember, however, that role models are not infallible, and they are still capable of making silly mistakes. How they respond to a blunder, however, can help provide new insight into how you go about tackling your own. Especially as adults, we should recognise when someone we like crosses a line, and hold them accountable rather than emulate their behaviour or parrot any ridiculous rhetoric.

And while it's good to have, say, your gramps, Mo Farah or Luke Skywalker as lifelong role models, try not to fall into the trap of measuring their successes and victories against your own experiences. Life can feel like a race, but your only opponent is yourself – and it's unlikely you're going to blow up the Death Star anytime soon.

Comparison is the thief of joy
Why you should focus on what you have and not the success of others

It's an all-too-easy trap to fall into, but you should not compare your life with that of friends, family, peers and celebrities you aspire to be like. You will only take the wind out of your own achievements and leave yourself wanting more when you should be celebrating or feeling satisfied. Everyone is different, and it is likely that you're only comparing yourself to a distorted highlight reel that has all the bad stuff filtered out. Instead of wasting energy on this, try practising gratitude. Find some time to jot down three things you are grateful for at that particular moment. The list might seem insignificant to begin with, but keep adding to it. When you return to it when it's bursting with positive things you enjoy, it will feel all the more rewarding and serve as a reminder of the good things you have in life.

Knowing your role models

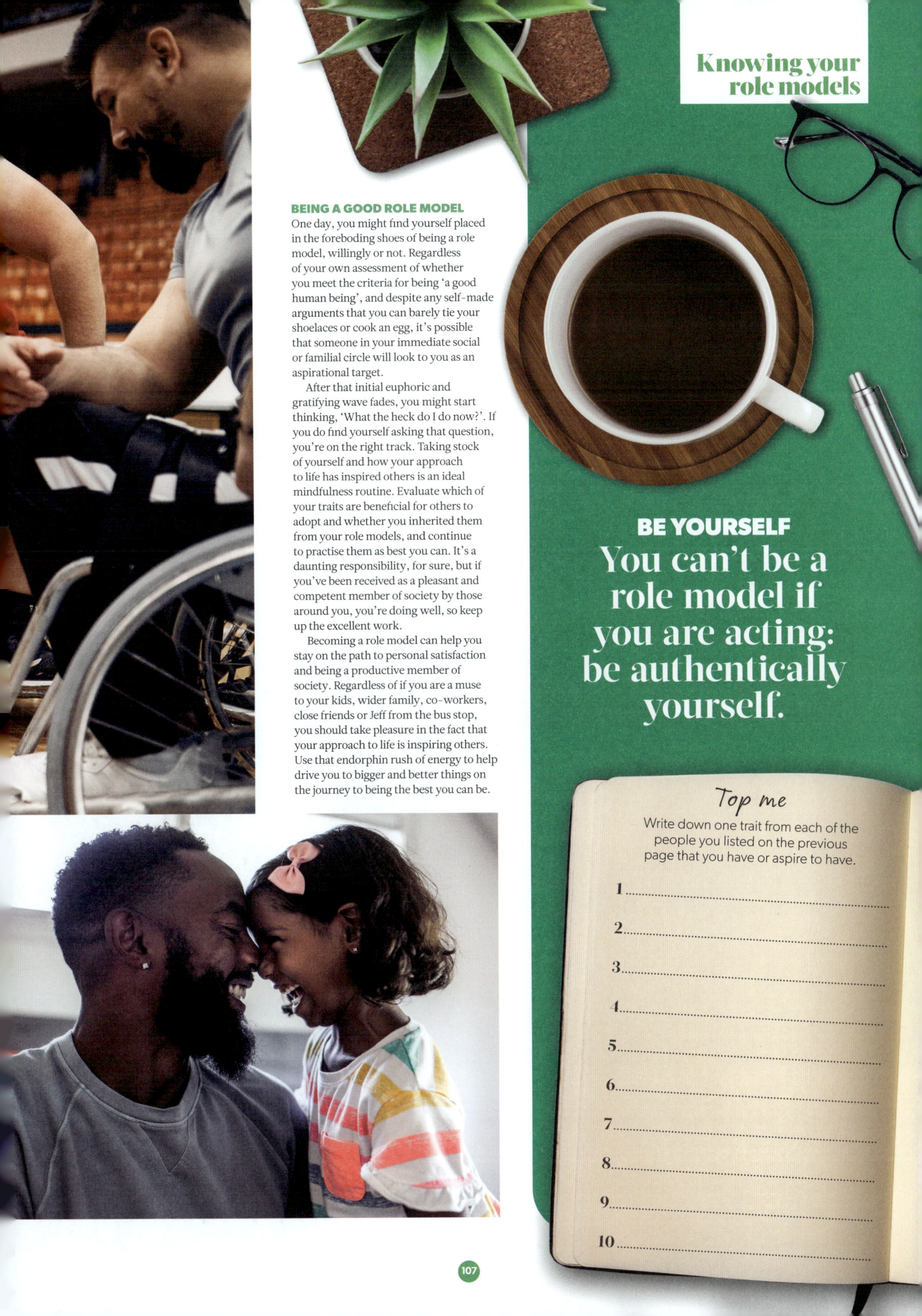

BEING A GOOD ROLE MODEL

One day, you might find yourself placed in the foreboding shoes of being a role model, willingly or not. Regardless of your own assessment of whether you meet the criteria for being 'a good human being', and despite any self-made arguments that you can barely tie your shoelaces or cook an egg, it's possible that someone in your immediate social or familial circle will look to you as an aspirational target.

After that initial euphoric and gratifying wave fades, you might start thinking, 'What the heck do I do now?'. If you do find yourself asking that question, you're on the right track. Taking stock of yourself and how your approach to life has inspired others is an ideal mindfulness routine. Evaluate which of your traits are beneficial for others to adopt and whether you inherited them from your role models, and continue to practise them as best you can. It's a daunting responsibility, for sure, but if you've been received as a pleasant and competent member of society by those around you, you're doing well, so keep up the excellent work.

Becoming a role model can help you stay on the path to personal satisfaction and being a productive member of society. Regardless of if you are a muse to your kids, wider family, co-workers, close friends or Jeff from the bus stop, you should take pleasure in the fact that your approach to life is inspiring others. Use that endorphin rush of energy to help drive you to bigger and better things on the journey to being the best you can be.

BE YOURSELF
You can't be a role model if you are acting: be authentically yourself.

Top me
Write down one trait from each of the people you listed on the previous page that you have or aspire to have.

1. ....
2. ....
3. ....
4. ....
5. ....
6. ....
7. ....
8. ....
9. ....
10. ....

Mindfulness for Men

BEST INTE

We all set goals, but goals can be difficult to achieve if we view them as an endpoint and not as a manifestation of ongoing change in our lives

Goals help you to stay focused. Everyday life is full of noise and a seemingly never-ending list of things that need to get done. We all know how easy it is to get distracted with small jobs that crop up screaming for attention, and then the larger pieces of work – without deadlines – get missed. In fighting those fires, we lose sight of what is really important.

Often it can feel like your 'must-do' list is cluttered with things that aren't helping you grow. When we set a goal, and achieve it, our self confidence increases, and we find ourselves progressing towards that ongoing change we're committing to.

When we set goals, we can also map out our steps to achieve the result we're looking for; this helps to keep us on the right path and meet the deadlines we set ourselves. When setting a goal or an intention, it can be beneficial to share them with people close to you – as well as helping you with accountability, you might find you get some extra help from unexpected sources (or at the very least, you'll be showing others what you're focusing on).

NTIONS

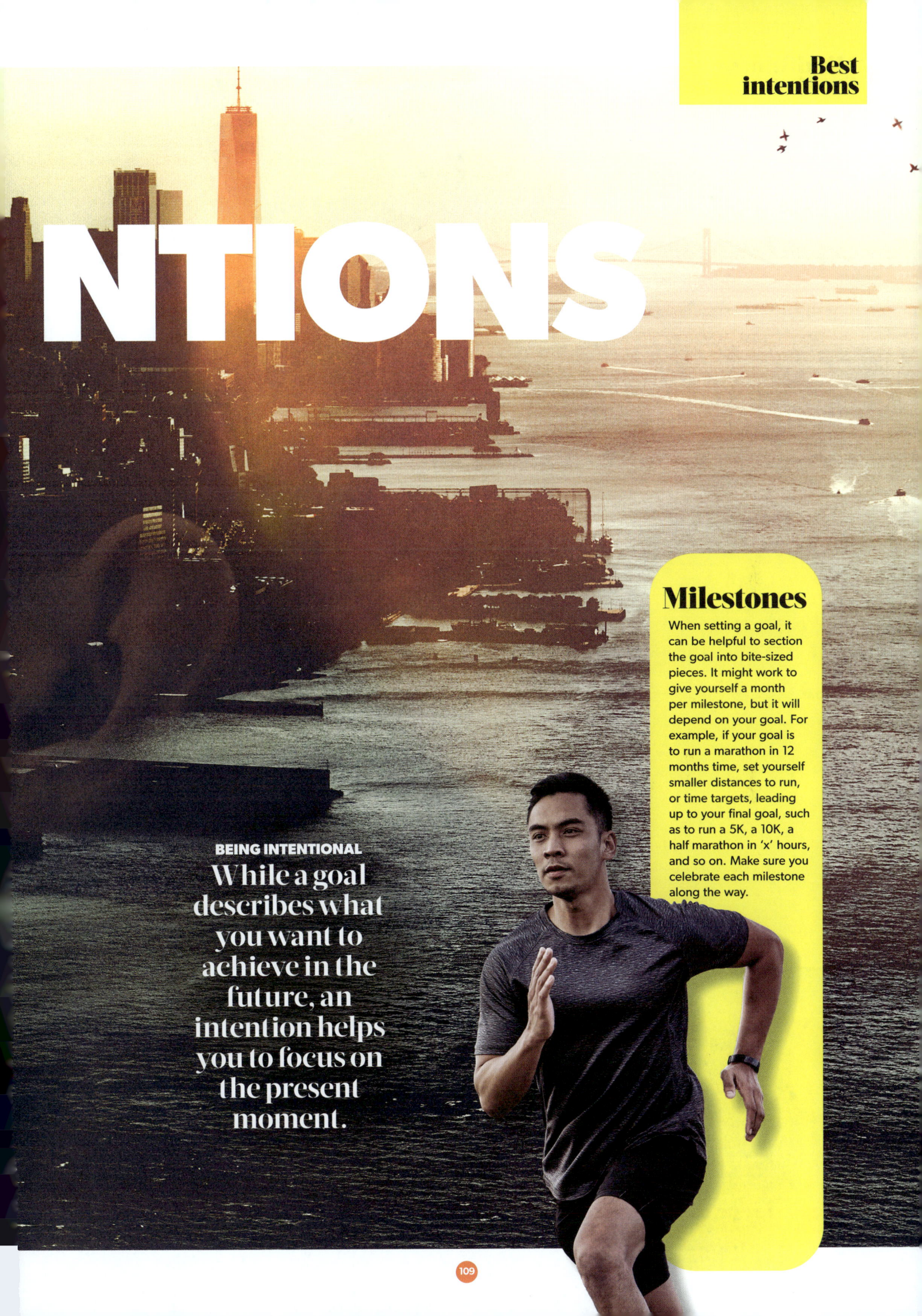

Best intentions

BEING INTENTIONAL
While a goal describes what you want to achieve in the future, an intention helps you to focus on the present moment.

Milestones

When setting a goal, it can be helpful to section the goal into bite-sized pieces. It might work to give yourself a month per milestone, but it will depend on your goal. For example, if your goal is to run a marathon in 12 months time, set yourself smaller distances to run, or time targets, leading up to your final goal, such as to run a 5K, a 10K, a half marathon in 'x' hours, and so on. Make sure you celebrate each milestone along the way.

Mindfulness for Men

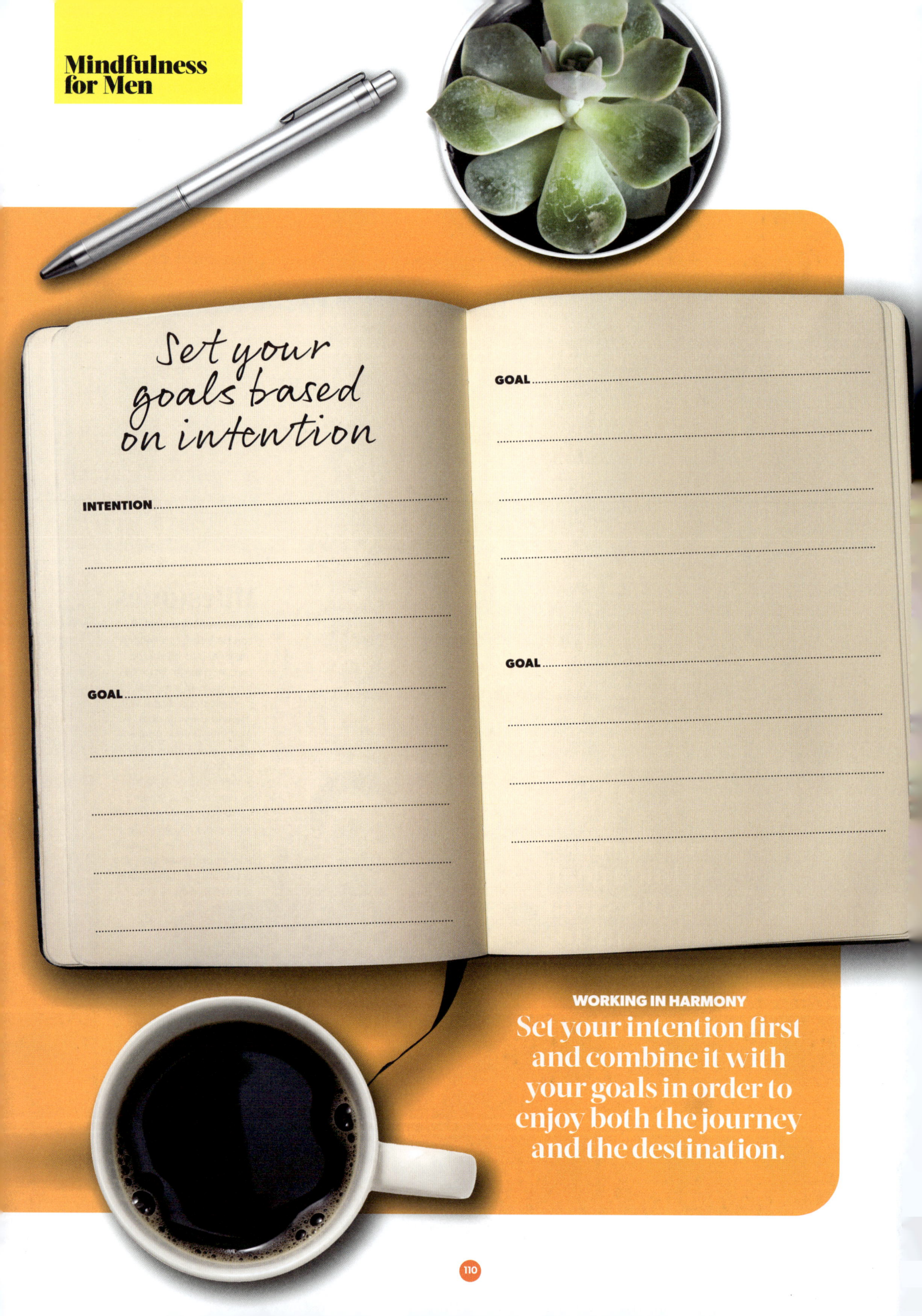

Set your goals based on intention

INTENTION............

GOAL............

GOAL............

GOAL............

WORKING IN HARMONY
Set your intention first and combine it with your goals in order to enjoy both the journey and the destination.

Best intentions

KEEPING POSITIVE
Our emotions impact our performance at work, school and home. When we use goals and intentions, we're staying positive in what we wish to achieve, and we're also setting out easily digestible steps, setting ourselves up not to fail but to succeed.

It is important to remember that stumbling on your goals shouldn't feel like a personal failure. We're all human and it is important to treat ourselves with kindness; mindfully reflect on what caused the 'failure' and how you can turn it around – could you have prepared more thoroughly? Did you get distracted by other projects? Keep digging down into the 'why' and you'll find the root cause of the problem. If you find yourself spiralling, take a moment to breathe and take notice of your breath and your body. Speak to yourself as you would a friend and resolve to try again.

INTENTIONS
Intentions are fascinating; they might feel like wishful thinking as you're putting pen to paper to jot down what you're working towards, but this act of articulating what you want and how you want to feel is a good way to develop your direction in life and towards your goals. If you struggle with having too many ideas and goals, setting an intention might help clarify what is really important to you. Many of your disparate goals may have the same root intention.

When setting an intention, take it slowly and listen to the voice inside your head. An intention is who you really are (without all those external influences) and also a good reflection of who you want to be. Intentions should be positive and a statement on how you want to exist in the world. Try to begin with an 'I' statement that backs up your goal.

TERMS FOR GOALS
A short-term goal is something to shoot for in the near future (generally under a year), and can be anything from journalling every day, waking up earlier, networking more, reducing your debt, or organising your work desk regularly. We use short-term goals for quick wins and quick feedback – you can see very easily if your methods are working. Long-term goals are a future accomplishment; they usually require lots of planning, and are normally achieved a few years in the future. Try to stick with one long-term goal, because setting too many can lead to not achieving anything. If the difference between a long-term and short-term goal isn't clear, think of your long-term goal as a life-long dream – there's no realistic way to achieve this in a week, so don't beat yourself up if you haven't given that TedTalk by next month!

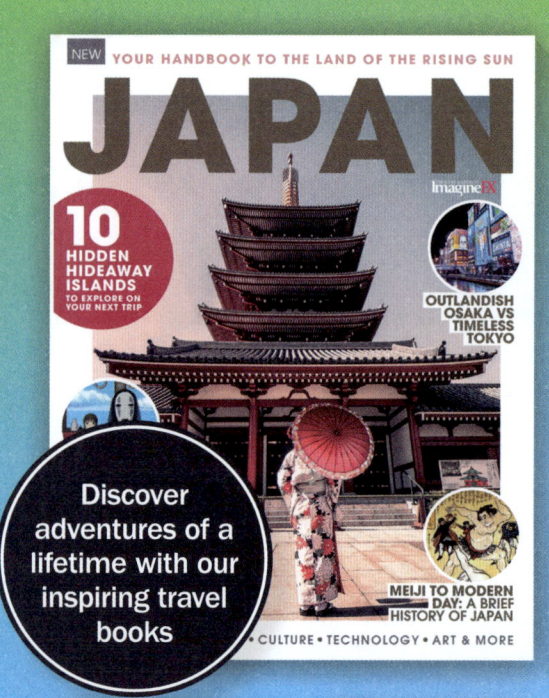

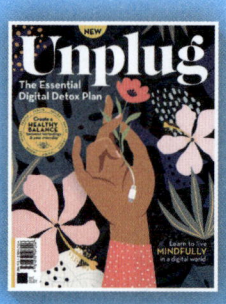

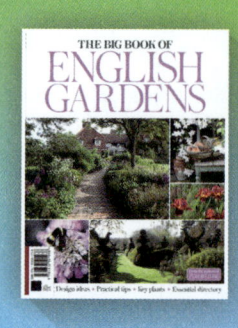

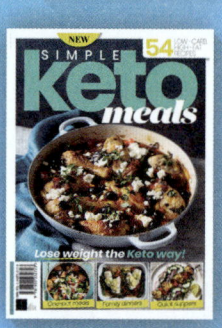

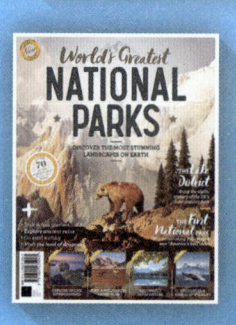

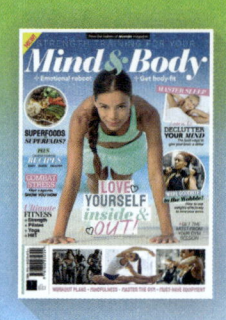

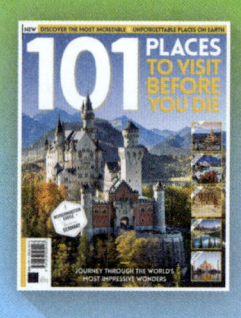

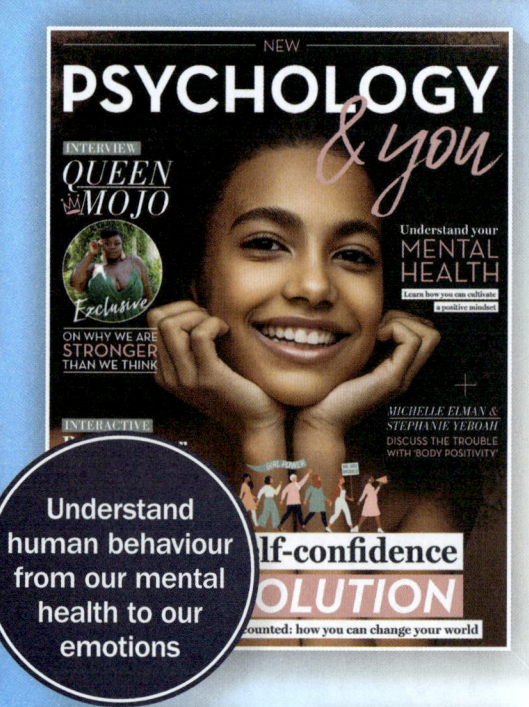

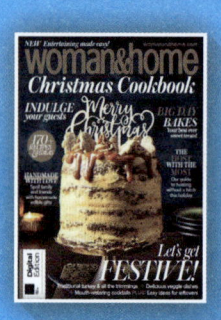

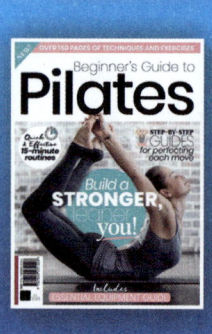

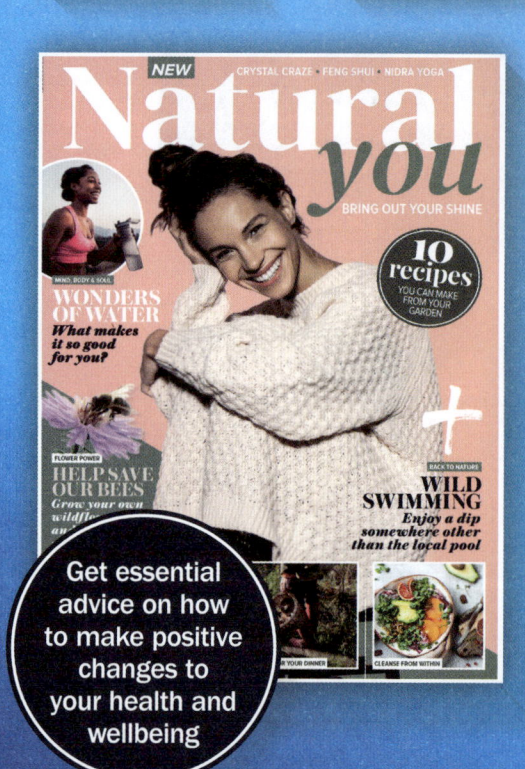

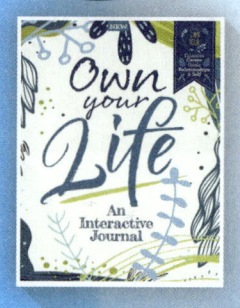

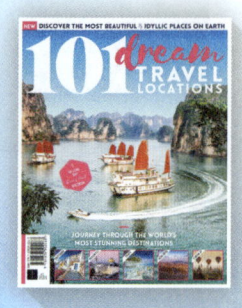

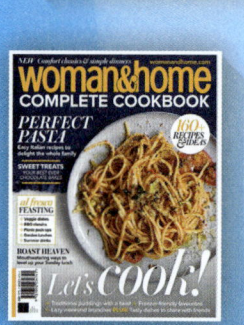

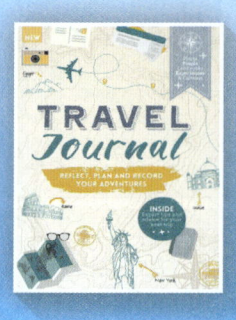

Discover adventures of a lifetime with our inspiring travel books

Understand human behaviour from our mental health to our emotions

Get essential advice on how to make positive changes to your health and wellbeing

✓ Get great savings when you buy direct from us

✓ 1000s of great titles, many not available anywhere else

✓ World-wide delivery and super-safe ordering

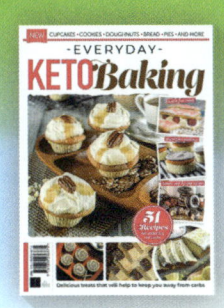

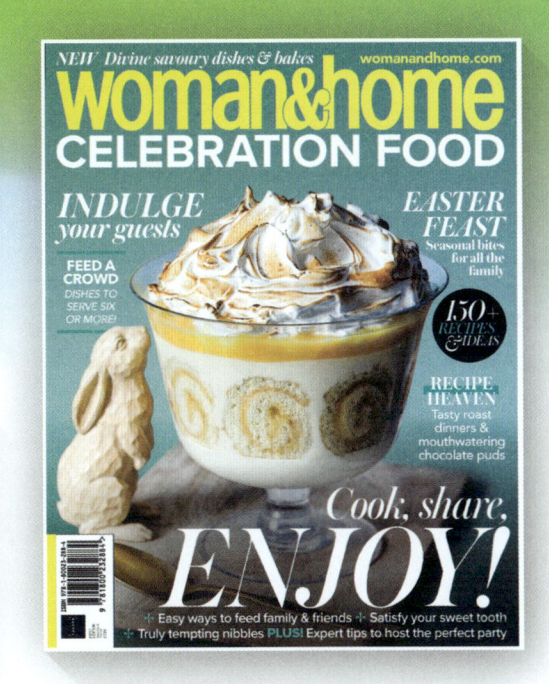

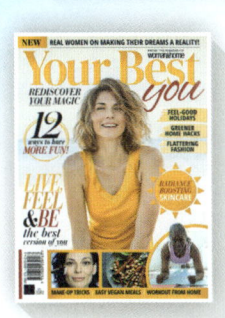

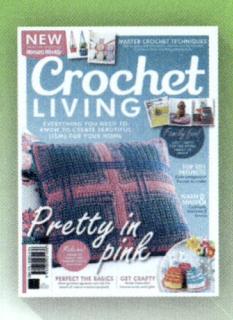

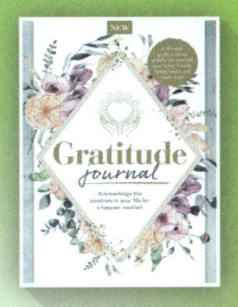

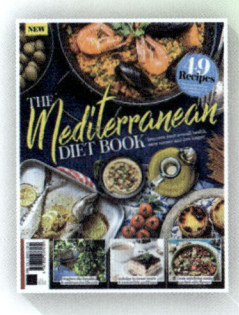

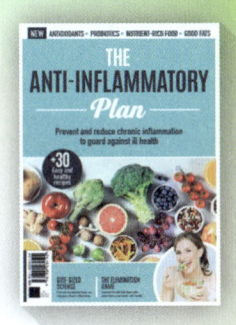

INSPIRING READS FOR A HAPPIER YOU

From travel and food to mindfulness and fitness, discover motivational books to enrich and enhance your life

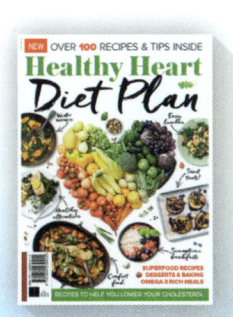

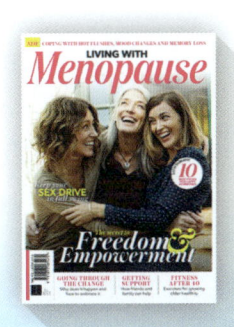

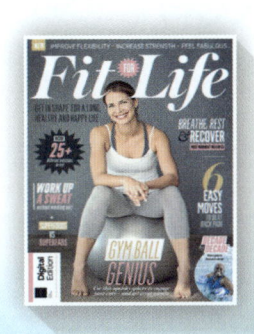

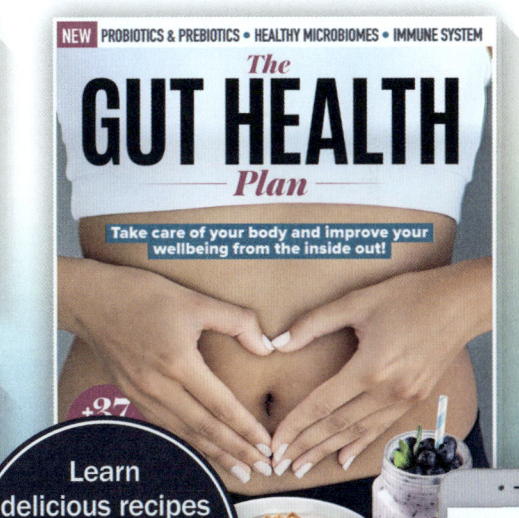

Learn delicious recipes and nutritional information for all tastes and lifestyles

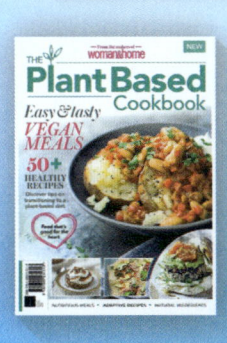

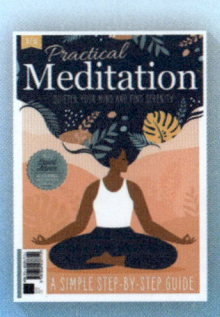

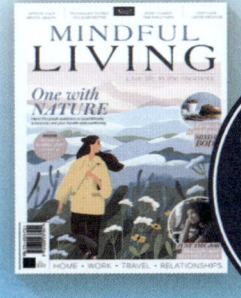

Follow us on Instagram @futurebookazines

www.magazinesdirect.com

Magazines, back issues & bookazines.

MINDFULNESS For Men

Future PLC Quay House, The Ambury, Bath, BA1 1UA

Editorial
Group Editor **Sarah Bankes**
Senior Designer **Perry Wardell-Wicks**
Compiled by **Dan Peel & Perry Wardell-Wicks**
Head of Art & Design **Greg Whitaker**
Editorial Director **Jon White**
Managing Director **Grainne McKenna**

Contributors
Edoardo Albert, Julie Bassett, Jo Cole, David Crookes, Aiden Dalby, Laura Mears, Laurie Newman, Dan Peel, Drew Sleep, Vanessa Thorpe

Cover images
Getty Images

Photography
All copyrights and trademarks are recognised and respected

Advertising
Media packs are available on request
Commercial Director **Clare Dove**

International
Head of Print Licensing **Rachel Shaw**
licensing@futurenet.com
www.futurecontenthub.com

Circulation
Head of Newstrade **Tim Mathers**

Production
Head of Production **Mark Constance**
Production Project Manager **Matthew Eglinton**
Advertising Production Manager **Joanne Crosby**
Digital Editions Controller **Jason Hudson**
Production Managers **Keely Miller, Nola Cokely, Vivienne Calvert, Fran Twentyman**

Printed in the UK

Distributed by Marketforce, 5 Churchill Place, Canary Wharf, London, E14 5HU
www.marketforce.co.uk – For enquiries, please email:
mfcommunications@futurenet.com

Mindfulness for Men Second Edition (LBZ5808)
© 2024 Future Publishing Limited

We are committed to only using magazine paper which is derived from responsibly managed, certified forestry and chlorine-free manufacture. The paper in this bookazine was sourced and produced from sustainable managed forests, conforming to strict environmental and socioeconomic standards.

All contents © 2024 Future Publishing Limited or published under licence. All rights reserved. No part of this magazine may be used, stored, transmitted or reproduced in any way without the prior written permission of the publisher. Future Publishing Limited (company number 2008885) is registered in England and Wales. Registered office: Quay House, The Ambury, Bath BA1 1UA. All information contained in this publication is for information only and is, as far as we are aware, correct at the time of going to press. Future cannot accept any responsibility for errors or inaccuracies in such information. You are advised to contact manufacturers and retailers directly with regard to the price of products/services referred to in this publication. Apps and websites mentioned in this publication are not under our control. We are not responsible for their contents or any other changes or updates to them. This magazine is fully independent and not affiliated in any way with the companies mentioned herein.

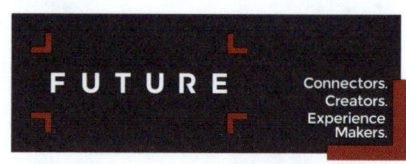

FUTURE Connectors. Creators. Experience Makers.

Future plc is a public company quoted on the London Stock Exchange (symbol: FUTR)
www.futureplc.com

Chief Executive Officer **Jon Steinberg**
Non-Executive Chairman **Richard Huntingford**
Chief Financial and Strategy Officer **Penny Ladkin-Brand**

Tel +44 (0)1225 442 244